Strangling Angel

Reappraisals in Irish History

Editors
Enda Delaney (University of Edinburgh)
Maria Luddy (University of Warwick)
Ciaran O'Neill (Trinity College Dublin)

Reappraisals in Irish History offers new insights into Irish history, society and culture from 1750. Recognising the many methodologies that make up historical research, the series presents innovative and interdisciplinary work that is conceptual and interpretative, and expands and challenges the common understandings of the Irish past. It showcases new and exciting scholarship on subjects such as the history of gender, power, class, the body, landscape, memory and social and cultural change. It also reflects the diversity of Irish historical writing, since it includes titles that are empirically sophisticated together with conceptually driven synoptic studies.

Strangling Angel

Diphtheria and
childhood immunization in Ireland

MICHAEL DWYER

LIVERPOOL UNIVERSITY PRESS

First published 2018 by
Liverpool University Press
4 Cambridge Street
Liverpool
L69 7ZU

This paperback edition first published 2021

British Library Cataloguing-in-Publication data
A British Library CIP record is available

ISBN 978-1-78694-046-9 cased
ISBN 978-1-80085-658-5 paperback

Typeset by Carnegie Book Production, Lancaster
Printed and bound by CPI Group (UK) Ltd, Croydon CR0 4YY

For my mother,
Eleanor
1945–2016

Contents

Contents

Acknowledgements

My greatest debt of thanks is due to Dr Andrew McCarthy, School of History, University College Cork. Andrew has been an obdurate source of support and encouragement throughout the research process and this book would not have been possible without his unyielding generosity of spirit. Andrew was always on hand to advise on difficult decisions relating to the more sensitive aspects of this research and his deep sense of decency and humanity was brought to bear on the historical assessments afforded the principal actors who populate this work. My thanks also to Professor Virginia Berridge and Dr Donal O'Driscoll for the insightful observations they brought to bear on my research.

I am grateful to the staff of libraries and archives responsible for the maintenance of documents and manuscripts which inform this book. I remain eternally grateful to Kieran Burke and staff of the Local Studies Department, Cork Central Library and to the many archivists and librarians at the Wellcome Archives & Manuscripts Library, London, who made my visits there simultaneously pleasant and rewarding. Productive visits to the National Archives of Ireland, the Royal College of Physicians Ireland, Cork City & County Archives, and the Boole Library & Special Collections University College Cork were made all the more enjoyable by the conviviality of the archivists and librarians attached to these institutions.

I am indebted to Professor Geoffrey Roberts and Professor David Ryan who, in their capacity as Head of School of History, University College Cork, saw fit to appoint me as a tutor and subsequently as a part-time lecturer. In the absence of research funding, these positions were crucial in allowing me to undertake the research which informs this book. I am equally indebted to Judge Yvonne Murphy, Professor Mary Daly, Dr William Duncan, and Ita Mangan for their support. The College of Arts, Celtic Studies and Social Sciences, and the School of History, University College Cork, generously part-funded my participation at a range of national and international conferences which allowed for wide dissemination of my research. My thanks are also due to the Society for the Social History of Medicine in this regard. I was honoured to participate in and contribute to international conferences convened by the American Association for the History of Medicine and the European Association for the History of Medicine and Health where I was fortunate to receive insightful feedback and support from a plethora of accomplished medical historians. I am eternally grateful for their collegiality and generosity.

My thanks and gratitude also go to the team at Liverpool University Press for publishing this book and to my editor Alison Welsby for making the publishing process such a vigorous and enjoyable experience. I am indebted to the anonymous referees whose comments and feedback improved the work. My thanks also to Rachel Chamberlain and the team at Carnegie Book Production for copy-editing my manuscript and producing such a lovely end product and to Eileen O'Neill for assembling a comprehensive index. I am grateful to the National University of Ireland (NUI) for awarding me a grant under the NUI Publications Scheme.

I owe a huge debt of thanks to my family. To my Dad Michael, who is always supportive and who, along with my sisters Catherine and Simone, experienced all the highs and lows of the research process. My thanks, and all my love to my children, Sarah and Jack, who were a constant source of necessary distraction, and to my darling wife Rachel whose good humour, faith, and companionship formed the bedrock on which this work is built. Finally, I wish to remember my late mother, Eleanor, who passed away while I was writing this book. Mum was an ardent advocate for childhood immunization and retained my, and my siblings, immunization cards long after we entered adulthood. This is for you, Mum. Thank you.

Michael Anthony Dwyer

Introduction

UNICEF and the World Health Organization (WHO) agree that childhood immunization is one of the most powerful and cost-effective public health interventions.[1] In 2015, more than 116 million infants, 86 per cent of the global infant population, presented for immunization treatment with a DTP3 vaccine.[2] DTP3 offers protection against the often-fatal consequences of contracting diphtheria, tetanus and pertussis (whooping cough) and averts an estimated two to three million infant deaths every year. These figures make it difficult to argue with Stanley Plotkin's assertion that with the exception of clean water, no other modality, not even antibiotics, has had such a major effect on global mortality reduction and population growth.[3] In Ireland, 96 per cent[4] of parents present children for immunization treatment to protect them against the ravages of formerly rampant diseases such as diphtheria, measles, mumps, pertussis (whooping cough), polio, rubella (German measles), tetanus, tuberculosis, haemophilus influenzae B (Hib), hepatitis B, meningococcal C (Men C), and pneumococcal disease.[5] In common with most countries, the childhood immunization programme in Ireland was founded on the public health response to diphtheria. This successful intervention ensured that Ireland has remained diphtheria free for almost 50 years.[6] This is a significant

1   Unicef / World Health Organization / The World Bank, *State of the world's vaccines and immunization*, 3rd ed. (Geneva, 2009).
2   World Health Organization, 'Immunization, vaccines and biologicals', (Updated July 2015).
3   Stanley Plotkin, W. Orenstein and P. Offit, *Vaccines*, (Elsevier, 2008), 1.
4   Health Service Executive (HSE), 'Immunization uptake report for Ireland', *Health Protection Surveillance Centre*, Q4 2015.
5   Health Service Executive (HSE), 'Protect, Prevent, Immunise', (Last updated 13 November 2013).
6   Health Protection Surveillance Centre, http://www.hpsc.ie/a-z/vaccinepreventable/diphtheria/factsheets/diphtheriafrequentlyaskedquestions/

achievement considering diphtheria continues to appear annually in many
European states, albeit in much reduced numbers than in former years.[7]

Prior to the mass social acceptance of childhood immunization in the
1940s, diphtheria was one of the most prolific child killers in history. The
formation of a leathery membrane in the lower airways induced death by
suffocation and earned diphtheria the moniker 'strangling angel of children'.
It showed scant regard for social status and infiltrated Europe's royal palaces
as sinuously as her slums and hovels. For parents and children in nineteenth
and early twentieth-century Ireland, diphtheria represented the 'most dreaded
disease of childhood',[8] but for their modern-day counterparts, diphtheria has
been relegated to a somewhat obscure disease. Few Irish doctors have seen
a case of diphtheria, let alone treated one. In Ireland, diphtheria has been
consigned to history, and so too have the horrors and mass fatalities once
associated with it. But how was this achieved? Was active immunization
received with open arms by public health authorities, the wider medical
community, and the general public? This book tackles these questions by
undertaking the first historical examination of the issues that underpin the
origins of active immunization in Ireland. It explores the driving forces
that shaped the national childhood immunization programme, and those
that opposed them. In addition, it examines the complex social implications
attendant on the introduction of this mass public health intervention.

In 1936, American medical historian Henry Sigerist remarked that the
history of medicine is 'political history, social history, economic history,
history of religion, and what not'.[9] Despite Sigerist's observations, the
historiography relating to the history of medicine and health produced
during the twentieth century – and this is particularly evident in an Irish
context – represents a canon of work produced largely within a Whiggish,
historicist framework, and is concerned mainly with medical institutions
and their alumni. This doxographical approach to writing the history of
medicine served only to fulfil physicians' eagerness to present the opinions
and practices of their predecessors and as Brieger noted, became 'the
hallmark of history in the service of medicine'.[10] In response, or indeed as

7 In 2016, cases were recorded in Australia (8), Austria (2), Belgium (6), Brazil (4), Canada
   (1), France (8), Germany (9), Latvia (6), Netherlands (3), New Zealand (1), Spain (1),
   Sweden (4), and the United Kingdom (1). Diphtheria remains most prevalent in India
   (3,380), Madagascar (2,865), Indonesia (342), Nepal (140), and Myanmar (136). Source:
   World Health Organization, 'Diptheria reported cases' (updated 6 September 2017).
8 Department of Local Government and Public Health, *Third Report 1925–28*, 34.
9 Henry Sigerist, 'The history of medicine and the history of disease', *Bulletin of the
   Institute of the History of Medicine*, Vol. 4 (1936), 1–13.
10 Gert Brieger, 'The historiography of medicine', in Bynam, W. F., and Porter, R. (eds),
   Companion encyclopaedia of the history of medicine, Vol. 1 (London, 1993), 24.

a backlash against this internalist and positivist approach, the latter half of
the twentieth century witnessed the influence of post-modernist scholarship
and the conceptualization of disease as a purely social construct, and public
health as a purely regulatory mechanism.[11]

Notwithstanding the constructivist epistemological turn, many historians
of medicine and health have sought to situate their research in a broader
social context. In 1962, Charles Rosenberg's[12] evaluation of the political,
medical, and social responses to historical epidemics in New York City
not only informed readers about disease and medical knowledge at a given
moment in time, but as Brandt asserts, in the process, opened up virtually
every aspect of society and politics.[13] Rosenberg's approach went beyond the
'history of medicine' to produce studies which would be more accurately
described as the 'history of health'.[14] Historians who follow Rosenberg's lead
recognize that all medical actions are, more generally, interactions between
disparate social groups and that a broader historical gaze must be employed
not only to explore the great doctors and their discoveries, but to consider to
whom those discoveries were applied, and how they were received.[15]

Recent scholarship has led to an expansion of historical knowledge and
understanding within the public health profession. In relation to childhood
immunization, factors which determine levels of vaccine confidence continue
to attract interest from a range of academics in the fields of science, public
health, and anthropology, and while it is acknowledged that clear communication of evidence-based information regarding the benefits and risks of
vaccines is essential, it is equally acknowledged that communication alone
will not address the 'vaccine confidence gap'.[16] Anti-vaccination groupings
have been greatly 'aided and abetted' by the internet, an uncritical media,

11 For example, Michel Foucault (Translated by A. M. Sheridan), *The birth of the clinic:
    An archaeology of medical perception* (London, 2009) and Peter Conrad, Peter and Joseph
    W. Schneider, *Deviance and medicalization: From badness to sickness* (Philadelphia,
    1992).
12 Charles E. Rosenberg, *The cholera years: The United States in 1832, 1849 and 1866*
    (Chicago, 1962). See also, Rosenberg, *Explaining epidemics and other studies in the
    history of medicine* (Cambridge, 1992), and with Rosemary Stevens (ed.) *History and
    health policy in the United States: Putting the past back in* (New Jersey, 2006).
13 Brandt, Allan M., 'Emerging themes in the history of medicine', *The Millbank
    Quarterly*, Vol. 69, No. 2 (1991), 199–14.
14 For an excellent overview of the changing definitions of the history of public health see
    Dorothy Porter, *Health, civilisation and the state: A history of public health from ancient
    to modern times* (London, 1999), 1–4.
15 Judith Walzer Leavitt, 'Medicine in context', *American Historical Review*, Vol. 95
    (December 1990), 1471–72. See also, Judith Walzer Leavitt, 'Writing public health
    history: The need for a social scaffolding', *Reviews in American History*, Vol. 4, No. 2
    (June 1976), 150–57.
16 Brendan Nyhan, et al, 'Effective messages in vaccine promotion: A randomised

questioning of government authority and 'a misplaced belief that infectious diseases have diminished because of improved economics, environments, and use of antiseptics'.[17] However, in order to arrive at a more nuanced understanding of issues affecting vaccine confidence in a community, researchers must move beyond the reductionist pro or anti-vaccination labels to garner a more thorough understanding of a population's specific vaccine concerns, their religious or political affiliations, their socioeconomic status, and their historical experiences with vaccines.[18] Virginia Berridge has long argued that medical historians are well placed to offer 'long term and contextualised perspectives on current health issues'.[19] While Berridge cautions against any attempt to hijack historical scholarship in some misguided attempt to learn from 'the lessons of history', to find historical justification for policy agendas, or to support current activist points,[20] she is equally insistent that 'the historian of medicine and health is uniquely positioned to contribute to current debate, by providing context, and by bringing historical perspective to bear on present day public health policy issues'.[21] In relation to childhood immunization, the current public debate revolves around the question; *should* children be vaccinated? However, considering the World Health Organization assertion that 'diphtheria is a disease controlled by vaccines, but waiting to re-emerge',[22] this historical perspective may serve to contextualize the current debate surrounding childhood immunization, and to provide a visible, audible, and consequential explication of the reasons why we, as a society, opted to facilitate a mass programme of childhood immunization.[23]

This book draws on several historical fields. It is a history of the origins of childhood immunization; however, more broadly it relates to the social

   trial', *Paediatrics*, 3 March 2014. http://pediatrics.aappublications.org/content/early/ 2014/02/25/peds.2013-2365.full.pdf+html.
17 D. Gill, 'Vaccination, not vacillation', *Irish Medical Journal*, Vol. 104, No. 10 (Nov–Dec 2011), 294.
18 Heidi Larson, et al, 'Addressing the vaccine confidence gap', *The Lancet*, Vol. 378, No. 9790 (6 August 2011), 526–35.
19 Virginia Berridge, Martin Gorsky and Alex Mold, *Public health in history* (Open University Press, 2011); Virginia Berridge, 'History in the public health tool kit', *Journal of Epidemiology and Community Health*, Vol. 55 (2001), 611–12; Virginia Berridge, 'History in public health: who needs it? *The Lancet*, Vol. 356, No. 9245 (2 December 2000), 1923–25.
20 Berridge, et al, *Public health in history*.
21 Virginia Berridge, 'History matters? History's role in health policy making', *Medical History*, Vol. 52, No. 3 (May 2008), 311–26.
22 Unicef / World Health Organization / The World Bank, *State of the world's vaccines and immunization*, Part 2: Diseases and their vaccines: Diphtheria, 106.
23 In response to Richard Horton, 'The moribund body of medical history', *The Lancet*, Vol. 384, No. 9940 (26 July 2014), 292.

history of medicine, and addresses the paucity of historical scholarship relating to disease and the public health response in independent Ireland.[24] It engages with a diverse range of primary historical documents and aims to produce a nuanced account of the introduction and reception of active immunization in Ireland. Annual reports compiled by the Chief Medical Officers of Health for Dublin and Cork give a frontline account of the challenges faced by municipal public health authorities in their efforts to control diphtheria in urban centres. These rich historical documents have not previously featured in studies relating to Irish medical history and will inform the first study of health service provision from the perspective of municipal medical officers of health in independent Ireland. The annual reports of the Department of Local Government and Public Health reveal how the successes or failures of local initiatives influenced, or impeded, the rollout of active immunization on a national scale. Analysis of contemporary writings, medical journal articles, and newspaper reports situate events in Ireland within international developments and facilitates consideration of the contested medical opinion surrounding the much-promoted benefits, and much perceived dangers associated with active immunization. An immense collection of documentary material unearthed in the Wellcome Archives and Manuscripts Collection, London, elucidates the close involvement of the British pharmaceutical company Burroughs Wellcome Ltd with the anti-diphtheria campaign in Ireland. These primary source documents take the form of personal and legal correspondences, laboratory reports, legal documents, court proceedings, reports detailing visits to Ireland, internal memoranda, and an unpublished manuscript. Thus, this book goes beyond a reliance on traditional and familiar sources by introducing, and exploiting, new and for the most part previously unused primary source materials.

Although it is not immediately obvious from the surviving statistical record relating to infectious disease in nineteenth and early twentieth-century Ireland, diphtheria was one of the leading causes of child mortality.[25] Issues relating to nomenclature, lacunae in medical knowledge, and a perfunctory system of disease notification ensured that diphtheria morbidity and mortality in pre-independence Ireland was grossly under-reported.[26] Following the establishment of the Irish Free State in 1922, the first home grown administration undertook an appraisal of public health service provision in the state and quantified the prevalence of the principal infectious diseases. The

24 Mary E. Daly, 'Death and disease in independent Ireland, c. 1920–1970: A research agenda', in Catherine Cox and Maria Luddy, *Cultures of care in Irish medical history, 1750–1970* (Basingstoke, 2011), 229–50.
25 Children: defined as those aged between 12 months and 15 years.
26 Anne Hardy, *The epidemic streets: Infectious disease and the rise of preventive medicine, 1856–1900* (Oxford, 1993).

investigation determined that efforts to implement public health services were seriously hampered during the revolutionary period, that levels of infectious disease were at unacceptably high levels, and that diphtheria in particular was endemic in every district. This prompted the re-constituted Department of Local Government and Public Health[27] to advocate the rollout of anti-diphtheria immunization schemes in Ireland along the lines of those pioneered by William Park, Abraham Zingher and the New York City Health Department in the early 1920s.[28]

Historians of medicine and health have variously analyzed the social, political, and medical responses to disease, and their influence in shaping public health services in nineteenth, and early twentieth-century Ireland. Although it is acknowledged that diphtheria mortality caused 'serious concern' in the 1920s[29] and that a pilot immunization scheme in Cork County Borough was 'particularly successful',[30] diphtheria and its centrality to the origins of the childhood immunization programme in Ireland, has lacked the historical attention it warrants.[31] The first task of this book then, is to recover diphtheria from obscurity. Not to establish the disease as a 'worthy' subject of study but to offer a rationale as to why Irish health authorities opted to embrace active immunization and to embark on a national programme of mass childhood immunization. Active immunization was the most radical public health intervention of its time and involved injecting a potentially lethal toxin into healthy children. Even a close examination of the statistical record relating to infectious disease in Ireland could justify the decision to introduce mass childhood immunization, particularly when health authorities in Britain rejected active immunization citing safety concerns.

The second task here is to establish the historical significance of

---

27 For in-depth analysis of the formation of the Department of Local Government and Public Health see Mary E. Daly, *The buffer state: The historical roots of the Department of the Environment* (Dublin, 1997).

28 Park and Zingher, 'The control of diphtheria', *American Journal of Public Health*, Vol. 13, No. 1 (January 1923), 26.

29 Diarmuid Ferriter, 'Local government, public health and welfare in twentieth-century Ireland', in Mary E. Daly (ed.), *County & town: One hundred years of local government in Ireland* (Dublin, 2001), 116.

30 Mary E. Daly, 'Death and disease in independent Ireland, c. 1920–1970: A research agenda', in Catherine Cox and Maria Luddy (eds), *Cultures of care in Irish medical history, 1750–1970* (Basingstoke, 2010), 233.

31 Childhood illness in Ireland has received relatively little historical attention to date. This situation has been addressed somewhat by the recent publication of Anne MacLellan and Alice Maugher (eds), *Growing pains: Childhood illness in Ireland, 1750–1950* (Kildare, 2013), which deals with tuberculosis, influenza, rickets, smallpox, ophthalmia, and falling sickness in children.

diphtheria. Historical studies relating to the public health response to diphtheria undertaken by Hammonds,[32] Hooker,[33] Hooker/Bashford,[34] and Hobbins[35] argued that the management of diphtheria played a critical role in the development of public health institutions and policies in America and Australia. Hooker takes it a step further with the assertion that the emergence of mass immunization was the premier factor in the radical refashioning of the epidemiological profile of developed countries in the twentieth century.[36] The global adoption of mass immunization during the twentieth century was arguably the greatest of all public health interventions, although mass immunization was not uniformly accepted in all jurisdictions, and its advancement was either enabled or restricted by local conditions. This book analyzes the introduction, reception, and application of childhood immunization in Ireland by examining how the rollout of a national immunization scheme was determined by a cumulative historical legacy of past social, economic, cultural, political and administrative processes, and the ambivalent, uncooperative, and sometimes obstructionist stance adopted by medical professionals.

The historiography relating to the first decade of Irish independence has argued in favour or against the assertion that Cumann na nGaedheal's tenure, 1923–32, was marked by a conservative attitude.[37] The Irish economy was inextricably linked to, and highly dependent on trade links with Britain, and political, legal, and medical administrative structures in the Irish Free State were the legacy of an imperial past. However, this book argues that in the case of public health administration and service provision, central health[38] looked not to London, but to New York for inspiration, and this

32 Evelynn Maxine Hammonds, *Childhood's deadliest scourge: The campaign to control diphtheria in New York City, 1880–1930* (Baltimore, 1999).
33 Clare Hooker, 'Diphtheria, immunization and the Bundaberg tragedy: A study of public health in Australia', *Health and History*, Vol. 2, No. 1 (July 2000), 52–78.
34 Clare Hooker and Alison Bashford, 'Diphtheria and Australian public health: Bacteriology and its complex applications, c.1890–1930', *Medical History*, No. 46 (2002), 41–64.
35 Peter Hobbins, '"Immunization is as popular as a death adder": The Bundaberg tragedy and the politics of medical science in interwar Australia', *Social History of Medicine*, Vol. 24, No. 2 (2011), 426–44.
36 Hooker, *Health and History*, 52.
37 For discussion on the historiological arguments see Jason Knirck, *Afterimage of the revolution: Cumann na nGaedheal and Irish politics, 1922–1932* (Wisconsin, 2014). For in-depth analysis of the Cumann na nGaedheal tenure see Ciara Meehan, *The Cosgrave party: A history of Cumann na nGaedheal* (Dublin 2010), John M. Regan, *Countering the revolutionaries: An examination of the Cumann na nGaedheal party 1922–25* (Belfast, 1994), and Donal Patrick Corcoran, *Freedom to achieve freedom: The Irish Free State 1922–32* (Dublin, 2013).
38 For abbreviation, the Department of Local Government and Public Health will be

becomes most apparent when examining British and Irish attitudes to disease prevention in general, and efforts to control diphtheria in particular. In her comparative analysis of the rollout of anti-diphtheria immunization in Britain and Canada, Jane Lewis argued that the delayed introduction of active immunization in Britain was due to economic considerations, and to a lesser degree to a diminished degree of initiative among the medical community.[39] Martin Gorsky challenged Lewis's interpretation by asserting that, as early as the 1920s, many local medical officers in Britain had embraced the system of anti-diphtheria immunization based on the American model, but their efforts were frustrated by the legacy of popular anti-vaccination sentiment and the absence of a strong lead from the state.[40] This book suggests that Irish health authorities promoted anti-diphtheria immunization along the lines of the American model and encouraged local medical officers of health to implement schemes of active immunization in their districts. Despite the persistence of the British medical model among the post-independence medical community, Irish public health authorities and municipal medical officers eschewed the reticence of their British counterparts, broke with Victorian concepts of disease control and embraced new public health methodologies in their bid to control diphtheria. However, the reception of new public health methodologies by the wider, more conservative, medical community in Ireland was marked by a pervasive sanitarian ideology, coupled with concerns relating to medical authority and traditional income streams: eliciting attitudes ranging from uncooperative to downright obstructionist.

Anne Hardy acknowledges that in the early twentieth century, popular responses to new preventive measures were not immediate, positive, or uncomplicated, and that historical interest has generally focused on the creation and achievement of the new, rather than the process of diffusion and acceptance in medical practice and patient culture.[41] With this in mind, this book aims to avoid the production of a purely teleological account of the triumph of bacteriology over disease. It argues that the necessary components required to implement a successful childhood immunization programme –

referred to as 'central health' throughout the text.

39 Jane Lewis, 'The prevention of diphtheria in Canada and Britain 1914–1945', *Journal of Social History*, Vol. 20, No. 1 (Autumn 1986), 163–76. Lewis's thesis is maintained in a more recent article by P. P. Mortimer, 'The diphtheria vaccine debacle of 1940 that ushered in comprehensive childhood immunization in the United Kingdom', *Epidemiology and Infection*, Vol. 139 (2001), 487–93.

40 Martin Gorsky, 'Public health in inter-war Britain: Did it fail?' *Dynamis*, Vol. 28 (2008), 91.

41 Anne Hardy, 'Review: Evelynn Maxine Hammonds, *Childhood's deadliest scourge: The campaign to control diphtheria in New York City, 1880–1930* (Baltimore, 1999)', *Medical History*, Vol. 45, No. 2 (March 2001), 297–99.

political will, public confidence, the cooperation of the medical profession, the availability of a safe and efficient anti-diphtheria prophylactic, and the existence of an administrative framework to oversee systematic public health service delivery – did not combine organically in an Irish context, but were forged through conflict and tragedy.

The opening chapter rescues diphtheria from obscurity, offering a rationale as to why Irish health authorities opted to embrace a new and radical public health intervention and why they set the eradication of diphtheria amongst the first of their national goals. A study of surviving statistical data relating to infectious disease in nineteenth and early twentieth-century Ireland does not suggest that such an intervention was warranted. However, despite the distinct lack of diphtheria notifications recorded in this period, this chapter will show that diphtheria was indeed a major child killer.

Chapter two will discuss how, from the 1880s, diphtheria increasingly became an urban disease in Britain, Europe and America,[42] and it is unlikely that Irish urban centres managed to avoid this ominous trend. The introduction of the Infectious Disease (Ireland) Act in 1906, and the mandatory obligation this legislation placed on local authorities to notify outbreaks of infectious disease, exposed the true prevalence of diphtheria in Ireland. The burgeoning, albeit reluctant, acknowledgement by local authorities in Dublin and Cork that diphtheria was endemic in their districts brought with it realization that a comprehensive public health response was required. Radical reform of public health administration and service provision in the newly independent Irish Free State, meant that Irish health authorities were well placed to take advantage of cutting edge laboratory-based measures to control infectious disease. It examines the development of anti-diphtheria antitoxin and its application as a preventive measure on a mass scale in New York in the early 1920s before considering how this radical public health intervention was received by health authorities and medical professionals in Britain and Ireland. This chapter will show how Irish health officials and medical officers eschewed the reticence of their British counterparts, readily abandoned traditional sanitarian approaches to disease control and embraced new public health methodologies in a bid to protect child life.

Chapter three examines the rollout of anti-diphtheria schemes in the Irish Free State. It argues that a successful – albeit small-scale – anti-diphtheria scheme undertaken in Dundalk, Co. Louth, in 1927 influenced the introduction of new legislation designed to accommodate the rollout of a state-backed national anti-diphtheria immunization programme. An overview of the national picture is complemented by more in-depth analysis

42 Hardy, *The epidemic streets*, 93.

of local initiatives implemented by 'front line' medical officers in Dublin and Cork. These case studies highlight the dissimilar results obtained by a frugal and limited intervention in Dublin compared with the more comprehensive mass immunization scheme implemented by public health authorities in Cork. This chapter suggests that Cork city was the site of the largest anti-diphtheria immunization scheme ever undertaken in Ireland and Britain, the success of which drew national and international attention.

Chapter four suggests that although the practical application of anti-diphtheria immunization in Cork achieved good results, its success was qualified somewhat by the limitations of Burroughs Wellcome's anti-diphtheria serum TAM. To reduce the occurrence of post-treatment diphtheria cases – occurrences which undermined public confidence in active immunization – field epidemiologist Jack Saunders introduced an experimental 'one-shot' Burroughs Wellcome anti-diphtheria antigen in Cork. This chapter explores the development of Burroughs Wellcome's Alum-Toxoid anti-diphtheria antigen and the relationships that developed between the British pharmaceutical company and Irish medical officers: the former eager to field trial experimental anti-diphtheria serums unrestrained by restrictive British legislation and the latter eager to embrace any solution, however radical, to leverage a modicum of control over diphtheria and its often-fatal consequences, even if this meant side-lining the rights of vulnerable children residing in state-run institutions.

Chapter five examines the Ring College immunization disaster, in which 24 children reportedly contracted tuberculosis and one 12-year-old girl died following routine anti-diphtheria immunization. The existing historiography relating to the Ring incident has, without exception, insisted that Burroughs Wellcome Ltd mistakenly supplied a bottle of live tuberculosis in lieu of a bottle of the anti-diphtheria serum toxoid-antitoxin floccules (TAF), even though this charge was not substantiated by a High Court ruling in 1939.[43] This chapter provides new evidence suggesting that liability for the tragedy

---

43 James Deeny, *To cure and to care: Memoirs of a Chief Medical Officer* (Dublin 1989), 189. Deeny states that 'through a mishap the children at Ring were injected with live tubercle bacilli'. Greta Jones, *Captain of all these men of death: The history of tuberculosis in nineteenth and twentieth-century Ireland* (New York, 2001), 157. Jones states that the immunization disaster was due to 'vaccine imported from Burroughs Wellcome contaminated by live tuberculosis'. Peter Hobbins, '"Immunization is as popular as a death adder": The Bundaberg tragedy and the politics of medical science in interwar Australia', *Social History of Medicine*, Vol. 24, No. 2 (2011), 426–44. Hobbins states that 'the TAF vaccine had been contaminated in the bottle before use'. Church & Tansey, *Burroughs Wellcome & Co: Knowledge, trust, profit and the transformation of the British pharmaceutical industry, 1880–1940* (Lancaster, 2007), 355. Church and Tansey assert that a former employee of Wellcome, R. A. Q. O'Meara stated that 'if he had been called to give evidence Wellcome would have lost the case'.

lay not with Burroughs Wellcome Ltd, but with the local attending doctor
and his advisors, who mounted a conspiracy to cover up initial negligence
in administering the immunization scheme and subsequent perfunctory
medical treatment of the affected children.

Chapter six argues that by the end of 1936, the Irish Free State had come
close to incepting an operational national anti-diphtheria immunization
scheme. This is a noteworthy achievement, as state-backed anti-diphtheria
schemes were not introduced as an intervention against this pressing public
health issue in the rest of Europe until 1938, and were only pursued with
any vigour when wartime conditions exacerbated the problem from 1940
onwards.[44] If it had progressed unimpeded, the Free State intervention
seemed destined to eliminate diphtheria, and to become the first established
national childhood immunization programme in Europe. However, the death
of Siobhán O'Cionnfaola in April 1937, and the subsequent controversy
surrounding the Ring incident, asked serious questions of active immunization and ultimately undermined vaccine confidence among parents,
practitioners, and politicians. This chapter will evaluate the impact of the
Ring controversy and the social, political and medical implications left in the
wake of the incident.

Chapter seven undertakes close analysis of municipal immunization
schemes in Cork and Dublin in the wake of the Ring incident and in the face
of impaired public health service provision attendant on wartime conditions.
It argues that the municipal anti-diphtheria immunization scheme in Cork
city was the only intervention mounted in Ireland or Britain to attain immunization rates comparable to those achieved in North America. In Dublin,
failure to organize a comprehensive immunization scheme facilitated the
recrudescence of diphtheria in numbers not witnessed since the pre-vaccine
era, and increased diphtheria mortality left parents with a difficult decision
to make: to present children for treatment to a compromised public health
service or to expose them to a rampant, virulent, and increasingly fatal
diphtheria infection.

This book is important as it is the first comprehensive study of the origins
of the childhood immunization programme in Ireland. It portrays Irish public

44 For analysis of the delayed rollout of anti-diphtheria immunization in Britain see Jane
    Lewis, 'The prevention of diphtheria in Canada and Britain, 1914–45', *Journal of Social
    History*, Vol. 20 (1986), 163–76. For a brief overview of the rollout of anti-diphtheria
    immunization in mainland Europe see, Beyazova, Sahin, and Yucel, Ben S. 'Age specific
    diphtheria immunity', in Ben S. Wheeler (ed.), *Trends in diphtheria research* (New
    York, 2006), 119–34, and also, European Centre for Disease 'A historical perspective',
    *Prevention and Control, Scientific panel on childhood immunization schedule: Diphtheria-
    tetanus-pertussis (DTP) vaccination.* http://www.ecdc.europa.eu/en/publications/
    Publications/0911_GUI_Scientific_Panel_on_Childhood_Immunization_DTP.pdf.

health authorities as being progressive regarding their willingness to accept and employ new public health initiatives, and importantly, it highlights how this attitude differed from the sluggish response of their British counterparts. The book explores the radical public health interventions which pitted efforts to achieve communal health against the rights of the individual. It presents a historical precedent where the actions of one medical practitioner undermined public confidence in the immunization process itself. In an era when childhood immunization is increasingly considered more of a lifestyle choice than a lifesaving intervention, this book may bring some historical context to bear on a current public health debate.

1

Aetiology of Diphtheria
in Pre-independence Ireland

The old public health was concerned with the environment; the new is concerned with the individual. The old sought the sources of infectious disease in the surroundings of man; the new finds them in man himself. The old public health sought these sources in the air, the water, in the earth, in the climate and the topography of localities, in the temperature of the soils at four and six feet deep, in the rise and fall of ground-waters; it failed because it sought them, very painstakingly and exhaustively it is true, in every place and in everything where they were not.[1]

Hibbert Winslow Hill, 1916.

The history of diphtheria is traceable to a period 'almost contemporary with Homer'.[2] References to 'malignant sore throat' among young children can be identified in the writings of the Greek physician Aretaeus who, in the first century C.E., described a condition, which he termed 'Egyptian' or 'Syrian' ulcer, as it was most prevalent in those countries. Aretaeus traced the spread of these ulcers to the thorax near the windpipe – which occasioned 'death by suffocation within the space of a day' – and lamented that 'children, until puberty, especially suffer'.[3] Macrobius Aurelius recorded an epidemic that swept through Rome in 380 C.E., when sacrifice to the gods failed to liberate the city from the ravages of the suffocating disease 'angina maligna'.[4] Macrobius's account of this visitation

1 Hibbert Winslow Hill, *The new public health* (New York, 1916), 8.
2 Daniel D. Slade, *Diphtheria: Its nature and treatment, an account of the history of its prevalence in various countries* (Philadelphia, 1864), 17.
3 Francis Adams (trans.), *The extant works of Aretaeus, The Cappadocian* (Boston, 1972), 12–14.
4 Macrobius, *Saturnalia*, 1, 10.

was contemporaneous with the Goth invasion of the Roman Empire, and in the period spanning the fall of Rome to the fall of Constantinople, references to 'malignant sore throat' and 'angina maligna' remain largely absent from the historical record.

In January 1517, an epidemic disease 'wholly unknown to medical men' appeared in Holland. While displaying similar characteristics to 'angina maligna', an attendant infectious inflammation of the throat was said to be 'so rapid in its course' that unless assistance was procured within the first eight hours 'the patient was past all hope of recovery [...] the threatened suffocation, at length actually produced it'.[5] Outbreaks of disease displaying similar epidemiological characteristics occurred in Paris in 1576 and in Naples in 1618–19, where 5,000 victims perished.[6] In Spain, the physicians Villa Real, Fontecha, and Herrera described in great detail and accuracy, the *garotillo* (croup), and *morbus suffocans* (suffocating disease), which prevailed throughout the Iberian peninsula between 1581 and 1611.[7] An outbreak of epidemic disease in the Northern Italian city of Cremona in 1747–48 killed at least 1,000 people, mostly children. The disease caused ulceration in the throat, making swallowing and breathing difficult, and many died of asphyxia. While undertaking autopsies on deceased children, local physician Martino Ghisi discovered that in every fatality, the respiratory membrane from the larynx to the bronchi was inflamed and covered in a white substance.[8] Ghisi recognized the paralytic phenomena associated with the disease, and his pamphlet *Lettere mediche del Dotto M. Ghisi*, published in 1749, is recognized as 'an important, knowledgeable, early account of diphtheria'.[9] Ghisi's position as a provincial doctor ensured that his observations found a limited audience and it was the appearance of the disease in Tours, France, in 1818 and the findings of the investigating physician, Pierre Bretonneau, which made the greatest contribution to contemporary knowledge of the disease.

Bretonneau's findings resulted from 'numerous researches in pathological anatomy', which, he pronounced, 'brought together the notions of modern

5 J. F. C. Hecker, *The epidemics of the Middle Ages* (London, 1859), 207.

6 R. T. Trall, *Diphtheria: Its nature, history, causes, prevention, and treatment on hygienic principles with a resúme of the various practices of the medical profession* (New York, 1862), 76.

7 E. H. Greenhow, *On diphtheria* (New York, 1861), 17.

8 George Kohn, *Encyclopaedia of plague and pestilence: From ancient times to the present* (New York, 2008), 80–81.

9 Carlo Castellani, 'La "Lettera medica" di Martino Ghisi relative alla "Istoria delle angine epidemiche"', *Rivista di storia della medicina*, 2 (1960), 163–88. See also, Edgar Hume, 'Francis Home M.D. (1919–1813), The Scottish military surgeon who first described diphtheria as a clinical entity', *Bulletin of the History of Medicine* (1 January 1942), 48.

times and those transmitted to us by the ancients'.[10] An epidemic imported into Tours by the military legion of La Vendée prevailed from 1818–20 and took a heavy toll on child life. In the village of Elcour alone, 42 children were lost from 40 households, demonstrating the extreme prevalence and severity of the infection.[11] Diagnosis had hitherto been attributed to the known diseases of scorbutic gangrene, malignant angina, scarlatinal angina, and croup, but reports of associated choking, and strangulation were 'new to the greater part of the practitioners, and upon its diagnosis and treatment, opinions were divided'. Following extensive investigation of symptoms among afflicted children, and 22 post-mortem examinations, Bretonneau and his assistant, Alfred Velpeau, observed that 'the material obstacle offered to respiration by the development of the false membrane always appeared to have been the immediate cause of death'. Bretonneau concluded: 'The more attention I have given to the study of the phenomena peculiar to this inflammatory condition, the more it has appeared to me to differ from every other by characters, which are proper to it [...], let it be permitted me to designate this phlegmasia by the name of Diphthérite'.[12]

In 1855, severe outbreaks of diphtheria occurred in Paris and Boulogne. In Paris, the disease attacked both rich and poor, 'carried off a large number of children [...] and seemed to fall with the greatest severity upon the children of the wealthy English residents'.[13] In Boulogne, it claimed the lives of 341 children, all aged ten years or younger, and by 1858, epidemic diphtheria prevailed in 31 French departments, with 9,042 reported cases resulting in 3,549 case fatalities.[14]

Nineteenth-century English medical literature and the popular press paid a particular flurry of attention to diptheria during 1859,[15] and reported it in terms of a biological weapon; another 'French disease' imported into England. Reports from the early 1860s suggested that the disease was prevalent in the south-eastern counties of England, especially counties close to the port town of Dover, which had long-established trade links with Boulogne, and the nearby port town of Calais. In Canterbury, less than

10 Pierre Bretonneau, *First memoir*, in Robert Hunter Semple (trans.), *Memoirs on diphtheria, from the writings of Bretonneau, Guersant, Trousseau, Bouchut, Empis, and Daviot* (London, 1859), 6.

11 H. J. Parish, *A history of immunization* (London, 1965), 118.

12 Bretonneau, *First memoir* (London, 1859), 20. Bretonneau's pupil Armand Trousseau would later change the designation from *diphtherite* to *diphtheria*.

13 Trall, *Diphtheria*, 78. The suggestion that diphtheria exhibited 'a manifest preference for the English at Boulogne' is reiterated by Greenhow, *On diphtheria* (New York, 1861), 2.

14 Trall, *Diphtheria*, 78.

15 Anne Hardy, *The epidemic streets: Infectious disease and the rise of preventive medicine, 1856–1900* (Oxford, 1993), 81.

20 miles from Dover, some of the 'first cases' of diphtheria were recorded in the practice of a Dr Rigden, during 1857.[16] However, it is clear from the writings of Fothergill, Short, Starr, and Home, that diphtheria was prevalent in England from a much earlier period.[17]

The 'Strangling Angel' in Ireland

In Ireland, the physician John Rutty related an outbreak of 'epidemic throat disease' during 1743, which 'might pass under the denomination of sore throats endemial to this country [...] but was of a species wholly distinct, being very malignant and fatal to children, and eluding the skill of physicians'.[18] During 1740–41, Ireland experienced a devastating famine, precipitated by a spell of unusually cold weather and exacerbated by wartime conditions attendant on the War of Jenkins' Ear (1739–48).[19] In his scholarly writings on medical history, Charles Creighton observed that the fevers attendant on the famine in Ireland were hardly over when 'the plague of the throat began among the children'.[20] Rutty observed that although few instances were reported in Dublin, the disease was prevalent in Wicklow, Carlow, Queen's County (Laois), Kilkenny, Cavan, Roscommon, Leitrim, and Sligo, 'carrying off incredible numbers, and sweeping away the children of whole villages in a few days'.[21] He opined that the smoke which hung over the city of Dublin 'corrected the morbid effluvia', and he relied on the accounts of country physicians to furnish him with a description of the disease. Rutty extracted the following account from 'a correspondent of mine in the country', one Dr Molloy:

> It is peculiar to children, and those chiefly from a month to three, four, five, six, eight or nine years old. They commonly for a day or two, or more, had a little hoarseness, sometimes a little cough; then in an instant, they were seized with a great suffocation lasting a minute or two, and their face became livid; they have frequent returns of these fits of

---

16 Trall, *Diphtheria*, 79.

17 John Fothergill, *An account of the sore throat attended with ulcers* (London, 1754). See also, Thomas Short, *A general chronological history of the air, weather, seasons, meteors, etc. In sundry places and different times more particularly for the space of 250 years*, Vol. II (London, 1749).

18 John Rutty, *Chronological history of the weather and seasons, and prevailing diseases in Dublin, during forty years* (London, 1770), 108–09.

19 The War of Jenkins' Ear, was a conflict between Great Britain and Spain that began in October 1739 and eventually merged into the War of the Austrian Succession (1740–48).

20 Charles Creighton, *A history of epidemics in Britain, volume II, from the extinction of plague to the present time* (London, 1894), 693–94.

21 Rutty, *Diseases in Dublin*, 109.

suffocation like asthmatic persons. The said suffocation is ever followed by one symptom, which continues till they die, viz. a prodigious rattling in the upper part of the aspera arteria [windpipe] resembling that sound, which attends colds when there is phlegm that cannot be got up. It is scarce sensible when they are awake but very great when they are asleep. Their death is generally sudden, and when least expected. Many die in twenty-four hours, none live above five days.[22]

Molloy's account of 'epidemic sore throat' in Ireland during 1743 predates Fothergill's account of 'sore throat attended with ulcers' in London by four years. Thomas Short, through anonymous correspondence from 'an ingenious physician', claimed that an outbreak of 'epidemic sore throat' during 1743 had 'been carried from Ireland into Scotland'. However, it is clear from the records of the Medical Society of London that 'putrid sore throat' was widespread in England and Scotland in 1742; a visitation which claimed the lives of both sons of then Prime Minister, Henry Pelham.[23]

In 1842, for the first time, the Registrar General of England classified diphtheria separately as a cause of death[24] in Ireland it was recorded as such from 1864. However, until the identification of the specific 'diphtheria germ' by Edwin Klebs in 1883,[25] and the discovery of an accompanying potent toxin by Roux and Yersin in 1888, diphtheria continued to be mistakenly diagnosed and recorded, and was widely believed to be 'not contagious [...] as no reliable evidence has otherwise been given'.[26] In 1859, an unidentified medical doctor writing in the *Cork Examiner* claimed that diphtheria was simply 'a new-fangled name for an old-fashioned disease, malignant quinsy, which, in the days of our grandmothers, was successfully treated by emetics and bark'.[27] Similarly, in April 1861, a synopsis of an article from the *Athenaeum* advised that diphtheria was not 'a new disease' and 'that it attacks the wealthy in well-furnished, well-drained houses as well as the poor [...] it is communicable [...] it attacks families; but it is not highly contagious'.[28]

22 Rutty, *Diseases in Dublin*, 110–12.
23 Short, *A general chronological history of the air*, 306. *Memoirs of the Medical Society of London*, Volume I (London, 1787), 458. See also, Horace Walpole, *Letters of Horace Walpole, Earl of Oxford, to Sir Horace Mann*, Volume I (London, 1883), 134.
24 Hansard, House of Commons parliamentary papers, *Fourth annual report of the Registrar-General of Births, Deaths and Marriages, in England*, 1842 [423], 83.
25 Derek S. Linton, *Emil von Behring: Infectious disease, immunology, serum therapy* (Philadelphia, 2005), 70.
26 *Annual Report of the City Inspector of New York for 1860* as quoted in Frederick S. Crum, 'A statistical study of diphtheria', *American Journal of Public Health*, Vol. VII, No. 5 (May 1917), 445.
27 *Cork Examiner*, 21 January 1859.
28 *Cork Examiner*, 17 April 1861.

From its designation as a separate cause of death in 1864, diphtheria and its causation aroused increased speculation from medical and non-medical sources alike. In April 1864, an *Irish Times* correspondent sought advice on an assertion in Charles Dickens's *All the year round* that the cause of diphtheria lay in 'the modern-day custom of wearing low turn down collars instead of the old stiff white walls, which now mark so conspicuously the middle-aged man'.[29] Dickens's article asserted that:

> The national throat, guarded for so many centuries by ropes of muslin, black velvet solitaires, lace collars, and other knick-knack, was suddenly stripped of its defences, and thrown open to all the rude winds of the English year. The result blossoms out in the disagreeable form of diphtheria, nature's terrible warning of the danger and simultaneous correction of the folly.[30]

An anonymous contributor to the *Irish Times* countered the fashionista argument by asserting that adult males rarely contracted diphtheria, and that 'the modern fashion of turn down collars had no influence in producing the disease'. This contributor suggested that the increased prevalence of diphtheria was 'Doubtless, one of a numerous class of typhoid diseases, which act powerfully on impaired constitution, either by direct or atmospheric influence [...] and so impregnates the atmosphere with poisonous matter'. Furthermore, his own 'long held belief' was that electricity was the 'principal agent in the engendering of disease' and that in most epidemics, 'a disturbed state of the electric fluid in the atmosphere, and on the earth's surface will be found'.[31]

The 'miasma' theory of disease causation, more commonly referred to as 'the Great Stink' in urban centres, featured regularly in nineteenth-century public health reports.[32] In his *Report on the health of Dublin for the four weeks ending January 27 1866*, E. D. Mapother reported that 93 deaths were produced by whooping cough, croup, diphtheria, and convulsions, diseases which he insisted 'are usually excited by the breathing of tainted atmosphere'.[33] Similarly, a Local Government Board report for 1875 expanded on those circumstances under which 'enteric fevers including diphtheria were found prevailing' and focused on districts marred by

---

29 Charles Dickens (ed.), 'A Grumble', *All the year round*, 19 March 1864, 136–38.
30 Dickens, *All the year round*, 1864, 136–38.
31 *Irish Times*, 26 April 1864.
32 Stephen Halliday, 'Death and miasma in Victorian London: an obstinate belief', *British Medical Journal*, Vol. 323 (22 December 2001), 1469–71. See also Joseph Robins, *The miasma: Epidemic and panic in nineteenth-century Ireland* (Dublin, 1995).
33 *Irish Times*, 6 February 1866.

insufficient water supply, foul streams, wells polluted by soakage, wells polluted by surface drainage, accumulations of excrement, piggeries, dung heaps, open cesspools, porous soil saturated by sewage, and overcrowded housing conditions.[34]

Although the French readily accepted Bretonneau's findings on diphtheria, caution greeted them in Britain and Ireland. Anne Hardy asserts that Bretonneau's ideas went unheeded until a markedly virulent form of diphtheria appeared throughout Britain during 1858: prompting a *volte-face* from the medical profession, both on diagnosis and treatment.[35] Until the introduction of anti-diphtheria serum therapy in the late 1890s, physicians remained largely powerless when faced with diphtheria. Parents and physicians alike 'were tortured by the sight of children dying in an agonising struggle for breath, as the diphtheric membrane appeared to slowly choke them'.[36] In his novel *L'education sentimentale*, published in 1869, Gustav Flaubert paints a vivid picture of a young boy afflicted with diphtheria and his 'agonising struggle for breath':

> The child started to pull the linen bandage from his neck as if he wished to remove the obstacle, which was choking him, and he scratched the wall, clutching at the curtains round his little bed, looking for something to hold on to, to help him breathe. His face was bluish now, and all his body, soaked by a cold sweat, seemed to become thinner. His haggard eyes fastened on his mother in terror. He threw his arms around her and clung to her in desperation [...] The spasms in his chest threw him forward, as though they would break him. Finally, he vomited something strange, which resembled a tube of parchment. What was it? His mother imagined that he had brought up part of his gut. But he was breathing deeply, regularly [...] The boy was out of danger.[37]

In this case, which Flaubert claims to have witnessed first-hand, the boy appears to have coughed up the false membrane that obstructed his breathing. More generally, and only as a last resort, physicians were called upon to 'wield the knife' to perform an emergency tracheotomy. This

---

34 'Circular of the Local Government (Ireland) Board of August 1875 with memoranda thereon', *Manchester Selected Pamphlets* (1876) (The University of Manchester. The John Rylands University Library), 9.

35 Anne Hardy, 'Tracheotomy versus intubation: Surgical intervention in diphtheria in Europe and the United States, 1825–1930', *Bulletin of the History of Medicine*, Vol. 66 (1992), 536–59.

36 Hardy, *Bulletin of the History of Medicine* (1992), 537.

37 Gustav Flaubert, *L'éducation sentimentale* (Paris, 2000), 350.

entailed slitting the windpipe in cases where the false membrane seriously impaired the patient's ability to breathe normally. Hardy asserts that in Britain, 'tracheotomy had its advocates and its detractors', and with a success rate of between 25–30 per cent such operations were rare, and reluctantly performed.[38] Where a surgical intervention succeeded in bypassing the obstructed windpipe, there was no guarantee that the patient would survive. Fatalities generally ensued from excess production of diphtheria toxin, frequently inducing heart failure.

The absence of a satisfactory medical response to diphtheria resulted in a proliferation of remedies and tonics with dubious claims from treatment to cure. One of the earliest 'remedies', Morison's Vegetable Universal Medicine, was claimed to 'strike at the root of all diseases [...] and was found to be of invaluable remedy in the treatment of diphtheria'.[39] It was alleged of Scott's Celebrated Vegetable Pills that 'the public cannot obtain a safer or more efficacious medicine for the speedy removal of colds and diphtheria'.[40] Similarly, the makers of Holloway's Ointment and Pills professed that their product 'had been ranked before all curative agents' and 'soon affects a cure by judiciously removing diphtheria'.[41] Du Barry's Revelanta Arabica Food, supposedly effected '72,000 cures in cases which had resisted all other remedies', including cure 'No. 68,413', which Du Barry assigned to Pope Leo XIII.[42] Furthermore, Du Barry claimed its product 'restored perfect digestion, strong nerves, sound lungs and healthy liver', and promised to cure a myriad of afflictions ranging from heartburn to sore throat and diphtheria.[43] Brandreth's Pills, advertised as the 'great American purgative', were promised to produce, after a single dose, 'a wonderful change for the better' in those afflicted by colds, throat affections, and diphtheria. Brandreth's claims, that its product 'caused the system to throw off from the bowels and kidneys the impurities which were oppressing it', were supported by James Rea, Consul of the United States, who endorsed its introduction to Ireland in 1870.[44]

For those unable or unwilling to pay for a manufactured 'cure', the *Cork Examiner* offered some cost-free alternatives. It endorsed the advice of Dr Henderson of London, who recommended the external application of water to the throat, 'at degrees of temperature alternating from the highest human skin will bear, down to almost zero'. Henderson claimed to have successfully

38 Hardy, *Bulletin of the History of Medicine* (1992), 539, 542.
39 *Irish Times*, 25 June 1864.
40 *Irish Times*, 13 November 1868.
41 *Irish Times*, 8 September 1869.
42 'No more medicine', *Irish Times*, 5 July 1870.
43 *Irish Times*, 5 July 1870.
44 'Great American Purgative', *Irish Times*, 12 July 1870.

treated a number of diphtheria cases using this method and that he was 'prepared to verify his assertion by proofs'.[45] Another article promoting a remedy based on a West Indian treatment for diphtheria instructed the patient to 'take a common tobacco-pipe, place a live coal in the bowl, drop a little tar upon the coal, draw the smoke into the mouth, and discharge it through the nostrils'.[46] While such claims are patently dubious, the fact that advertisements for such products appeared in the local and national press on a daily basis highlighted both the lacunae in medical knowledge and treatment, and the fear instilled by the disease.[47]

The appearance of diphtheria in a community was rarely less than devastating, and its tendency to attack whole families exacerbated the impact. In 1859, a succession of 'close and severe family afflictions' befell the Tough family in Fyvie, Scotland. In December, Tough's daughter, Jean, died of diphtheria and in the following weeks the disease took the lives of his wife Ann, and his three remaining children, Mary, Christian, and James.[48] In Ipswich, shoemaker, James Gooding, lost three children to diphtheria in one week and became so distraught that he murdered his only surviving child, 'a little cripple girl, aged six years', before committing suicide by cutting his own throat.[49] In March 1863, five members of the Watkins family aged between four and nineteen years, contracted diphtheria and died over the course of 11 days in a small cottage in Swansea.[50] However, the worst recorded episode of diphtheria to impact on a single family occurred outside Londonderry in the town of Dungiven, where during November 1876, 'all eight children in one family died of diphtheria within seventeen days'.[51]

These tragic events, while devastating for families and their communities, received mere cursory mention in the press and medical periodicals. However, an epidemic outbreak of diphtheria in Germany among the Grand Ducal family of Hesse-Darmstadt concentrated minds in Britain and Ireland. On 14 December 1878, Princess Alice Maud Mary, Duchess of Saxony, Grand Duchess of Hess-Darmstadt, and second daughter of Queen Victoria, died from diphtheria.[52] Four weeks earlier, Alice's daughter, Victoria, developed diphtheria, and the disease subsequently spread to her four siblings and to her father, the Grand Duke Frederick William Louis

45 *Cork Examiner*, 5 January 1859.
46 *Cork Examiner*, 19 July 1865.
47 Tony Farmar, *Patients, potions and physicians: A social history of medicine in Ireland* (Dublin, 2004), 127.
48 'Heavy bereavement', *Irish Times*, 17 January 1860.
49 'Murder and suicide', *Cork Examiner*, 16 January 1864.
50 *Cork Examiner*, 15 April 1863.
51 *British Medical Journal* (22 November 1879), 827.
52 'Death of Princess Alice', *Irish Times*, 16 December 1878.

of Hesse-Darmstadt. Queen Victoria dispatched her personal physician, the renowned pathologist, Sir William Jenner, to Darmstadt to assist German doctors. Despite their best efforts, the four-year-old Princess Marie succumbed to the disease and died. While conveying the news to her surviving children, Princess Alice reportedly 'clasped them in her arms' and according to Disraeli, 'thus received the kiss of death'.[53]

Darmstadt prompted increased attention in the British press and medical periodicals, raising the profile of diphtheria and with it the realization that no remedy existed. Despite the efforts of 'the greatest English and German authorities' on diphtheria, the application of remedies 'which most recent scientific researches [sic] have discovered', failed to cure or arrest the spread of disease, and underscored the helplessness of medical science.[54] In accordance with the wishes of Queen Victoria and the English medical establishment, Dr Eigenbrodt, physician to the Grand Ducal family, and Professor J. Oertel, of the University of Munich, undertook a thorough investigation of the incident.[55]

Although it was not a rare occurrence for an entire family to contract diphtheria, Darmstadt prompted unprecedented attention, resulting in the most advanced set of clinical observations regarding diphtheria since Bretonneau's review in Tours almost sixty years earlier. Professor Oertel, in particular, produced an enlightened report on the tragedy, addressing the nature of contagion, the mode of dissemination, the characteristic 'diphtheritic process', the increased malignancy which accompanied propagation, and the different forms of diphtheria. In addition, he outlined detailed observations on the physical deterioration of the diphtheric patient, as well as an assessment of contemporary diphtheria remedies.[56] In January 1879, Oertel sent an English language version of his findings to the *British Medical Journal*, where he hoped that such a widely read periodical would inform others 'who have not so complete a knowledge of these conditions, and whose erroneous suppositions and conclusions may perhaps be thereby corrected'.[57]

53 A. G. W. Whitfield, 'The kiss of death', *Annals of the Royal College of Surgeons of England*, Vol. 61, No. 5 (September 1979), 390–92. In 1859, the twenty-two-year-old Queen Stephanie of Portugal also succumbed to diphtheria. See: *Irish Times*, 8 August 1859 and 'The late Queen of Portugal', *Cork Examiner*, 1 August 1859. Diphtheria also claimed the life of the Duchess Sophia of Bavaria, daughter of the King of Saxony in 1867. 'Bavaria', *Cork Examiner*, 11 March 1867.

54 'Lessons from the outbreak of diphtheria in the Grand Ducal family of Hesse-Darmstadt', *British Medical Journal* (4 January 1879), 15.

55 'Report of the medical history of the attack of diphtheria in the Grand Ducal family at Hesse-Darmstadt', *British Medical Journal* (4 January 1879), 6.

56 J. Oertel, 'The outbreak of diphtheria in the Grand Ducal family of Hesse-Darmstadt', *British Medical Journal* (11 January 1879), 36–39.

57 Oertel, *British Medical Journal* (1879), 39.

However, there is little evidence that Oertel's observations were accepted, let alone applied by British medical practitioners.

The slow acceptance of Bretonneau's designation of 'diphtheria' obliges a cautious reading of surviving quantitative data.[58] In England and Wales, the separate classification from 1838 onwards of croup and laryngitis from diphtheria ensured that former cases of scarlet fever became more easily recognizable as diphtheria.[59] As diagnosis improved, increased notifications of diphtheria fatalities were recorded, and a steady and gradual diminution of recorded fatalities assigned to croup, laryngitis, and scarlet fever ensued.[60] In fact, the increase in diphtheria morbidity and mortality in England and Wales was quite marked, rising from 95 per million of the population from 1859–63, to 253 per million of the population from 1891–95.[61]

It seems reasonable to expect that a similar trend would be evident in the statistical record relating to Ireland; that diseases formally classified as gangrenous sore throat, putrid sore throat with ulcers (angina maligna), scarlatina, quinsy, or croup in the first half of the nineteenth century, would increasingly become designated as diphtheria during the latter. Analysis of Irish mortality rates relating to scarlatina, croup, and quinsy reveals that between 1864 and 1900, mortality fell considerably, with no discernible rise detected in the incidence of diphtheria deaths.[62] Considering that at the end of the nineteenth century diphtheria was 'an endemic disease throughout the civilised world', its near absence from the Irish record is somewhat anomalous.[63]

In a letter to the *Irish Times*, Dr W. R. MacDermott, Poyntzpass, Newry, attempted an explanation. His father, Ralph Nash MacDermott, also a doctor and registrar of deaths, was aware of the term 'diphtheria', but like so many contemporary medical practitioners, he never used it. MacDermott argued that because medical texts published before 1860 did not use the word 'diphtheria', doctors trained and practicing between 1860 and 1890 did not commonly recognize the term, or record it as a cause of death.[64] He recounted an incident where he was called on to attend

58 Friedrich Loeffler, 'The history of diphtheria', in G. H. F. Nuttall (ed.), *The bacteriology of diphtheria* (Cambridge, 1908), 18.

59 T. Ridley Bailey, 'Public health progress in the Queen's reign, 1837–1897: being the presidential address of the Midland Branch of the incorporated Society of Medical Officers of Health 1897', *LSE Selected Pamphlets* (1897), 24.

60 Arthur Newsholme, *Epidemic diphtheria: A research on the origin and spread of the disease from an international standpoint* (London, 1898), 31.

61 Bailey, 'Public health progress in the Queen's reign, 1837–1897', 24.

62 Hansard, *Registrar General of Marriages, Births and Deaths in Ireland, Annual Reports*, 1864–1900.

63 Loeffler, 'The history of diphtheria', 16.

64 'The anti-toxin treatment of diphtheria', *Irish Times*, 26 April 1910.

to 'an able and well-read medical man' afflicted with diphtheria during the 1890s, who objected to MacDermott's use of 'the new-fangled term' diphtheria, even though it had entered the medical vocabulary almost fifty years previously. MacDermott acknowledged that 'diphtheria' was notifiable under the Infectious Disease (Notification) Act 1889, but he asserted that in Ireland, the term 'membranous croup' persisted as the most common term assigned to the disease.[65]

Addressing the Medical Society of King and Queens College of Physicians[66] in Ireland in April 1881, Derry-based physician, Walter Bernard, highlighted another reason why diphtheria remained largely absent from the statistical record. With regard to diphtheria, Bernard cautioned 'there are few diseases about which so many mistakes in diagnosis are made'.[67] He feared the misdiagnosis was so high that it was difficult, if not impossible to ensure that 'true diphtheria' was as common in a town as reported. Although he echoed Dr James Little's claim that 'diphtheria is rare in Dublin', Bernard asserted that 'diphtheria occurs in Londonderry, I have no doubt whatever [...] in my practice it has been my lot to treat many cases of this disease'.[68]

In his investigation into the prevalence of diphtheria in Britain, noted epidemiologist, Arthur Newsholme, corroborated Bernard's claim that diphtheria was most prevalent in Londonderry which experienced 'a rather large epidemic in 1889, followed by a still higher rise after an interval of two years in 1893'. Belfast, Cork, and Limerick County Boroughs were also adversely affected by epidemic diphtheria during 1893, though Newsholme observed that Waterford, and Dublin in particular, 'remained remarkably free from this disease' throughout the whole period.[69] The low overall incidence for a sparsely populated Ireland generally did not surprise him as he endorsed the hypothesis that diphtheria spread 'chiefly by personal infection'.[70]

Newsholme's correlation between the prevalence of diphtheria and population density make little sense in light of statistics he presented for Irish urban centres, as the most densely populated district, Dublin, recorded the lowest prevalence of diphtheria for the period under review. When compared with centres of similar population size in England and Scotland, Newsholme's population density argument regarding Dublin is even less

65 *Irish Times*, 26 April 1910.
66 King and Queen's College of Physicians in Ireland adopted the title Royal College of Physicians of Ireland under charter of Queen Victoria in 1890.
67 Walter Bernard, 'Diphtheria in Londonderry', *The Dublin Journal of Medical Science*, Vol. 71, No. 5, (2 May 1881), 402–04.
68 Bernard, *The Dublin Journal of Medical Science*, 1881.
69 Newsholme, *Epidemic diphtheria*, 48.
70 Newsholme, *Epidemic diphtheria*, 48.

convincing. Using the census enumeration of 1891, Newsholme recorded the population of Dublin as being 349,594. The urban centres of Sheffield (325,304), Manchester (351,189), Leeds (347,278), and Glasgow (397,673) lend themselves well to comparative analysis.

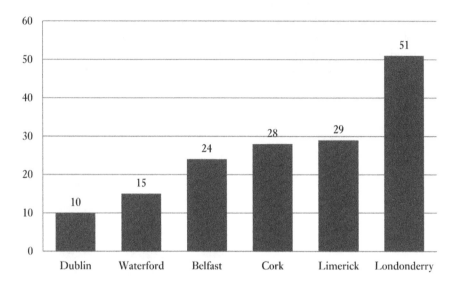

Fig. 1.1   Diphtheria mortality per 100,000 in Irish urban centres 1881–95.[71]

It is immediately clear that the notification of diphtheria deaths in Dublin was far lower than other urban centres of comparable population size, representing less than 50 per cent of notifications in Leeds, and less than 12 per cent of notifications in Sheffield. These figures suggest that the extraordinarily low rate of diphtheria recorded in Dublin should have attracted some close international attention. One *British Medical Journal* article acknowledged that the comparative exemption of Ireland from the diphtheria which has ravaged England 'is a striking fact, worthy of further consideration by epidemiologists'. However, that author was sufficiently happy to conclude that 'the small amount of diphtheria in rainy Ireland' confirmed the belief that 'the amount of diphtheria is greatest in the parts having the smallest rainfall'.[72]

When Dublin did come under some scrutiny, the infrequent notification of diphtheria in the city's pre-1898 health record became the focus of a more searching inquiry into the general activities of the city's health

71   Newsholme, *Epidemic diphtheria*, 48.
72   'Ireland', *British Medical Journal* (16 January 1904), 158.

authorities. As late as March 1900, public health officials maintained their claims that diphtheria was a 'very rare disease' in Dublin. Examined by Dr R. L. Swan, President of the Royal College of Surgeons, Dr John Day, Medical Superintendent to Cork Street Fever Hospital, stated that prior to 1898, diphtheria was 'largely absent' from Dublin with 'scarcely any cases coming in from the city [...] and few cases from the outlying districts'.[73] Dr Fitzgibbon, the long-standing medical officer to the General Post Office, concurred with Day, stating that for the years 1891–99, he had encountered only seven cases of diphtheria among the 1,600 post office employees under his care.[74]

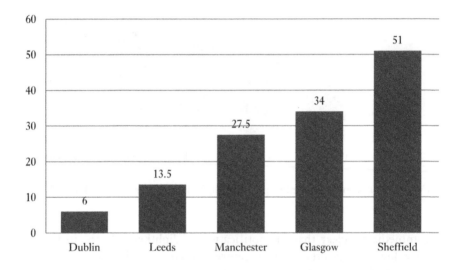

Fig. 1.2   Mean diphtheria death rate per 100,000 notified for the period 1859–89 for Dublin and urban centres of comparable population size.[75]

The complex nature of true diphtheria made it difficult to diagnose, let alone treat. In short, the disease confounded most physicians. It seems clear then that when diphtheria fatalities occurred, notifications remained hidden within a complex array of causes of death, obscuring its true prevalence. This

73 *Report of the Committee appointed by the Local Government Board for Ireland to inquire into the Public Health of the City of Dublin* (Dublin, 1900), 66. For an overview of the Dublin Public Health Inquiry 1900 see Lydia Carroll, *In the fever king's preserve; Sir Charles Cameron and the Dublin slums* (Dublin, 2011), 179–85.
74 *Public Health of the City of Dublin 1900*, 78.
75 Figures taken from Newsholme, *Epidemic diphtheria*, 29–48. As Newsholme presents the highest and lowest incidence of diphtheria for each urban centre, for purposes of comparison, the mean diphtheria mortality rates are presented here.

being so, it is reasonable to assert that diphtheria fatalities recorded during the nineteenth century are not a true reflection of mortality associated with the disease in Ireland.[76]

Know Thine Enemy

In 1900, William Langford Symes undertook an investigation into the symptoms and phenomena known as croup, and the detrimental effects that the designation had on the correct diagnosis of diphtheria.[77] Symes asserted:

> When sent for to a case of "Croup" we have no idea what lies before us. We picture a child choking from a disease perhaps beyond our control, or possibly it may be but a passing spasm. Between these two extremes an infinite variety exists. They are called "Croup", but the word practically only conveys that respiration is impeded in the larynx. We should be better off without the word [Croup ...] as deaths registered as Croup are mainly due to diphtheria.[78]

Analysis of registered child fatalities in Ireland for the ten years to 1896 reveals a myriad table of causes of death, which cloaked diphtheria fatalities.[79] In deaths recorded as occurring in infants, diphtheria is at number 35, registering 171 fatalities, whilst among children aged 1–5 years it is the nineteenth cause of death, registering 1,818 fatalities, together combining to account for an annual average of 182 diphtheria fatalities in children aged five years and younger. However, fatalities assigned under the denomination croup total 7,098 fatalities, or 708 fatalities annually among the same age groups. A consideration of these figures, in light of Symes's assertion that deaths registered as croup were mainly due to diphtheria, suggests that

76 Patrick Letters, 'Public Health and preventable disease in the counties of Cork, Kerry, and Waterford', *The Dublin Journal of Medical Science*, Vol. 107, No. 3 (1 March 1899), 181–89.

77 William Langford Symes, 'On the symptoms or phenomena formerly known as Croup; the diseases which produce them; and the clinical significance of the varied allied affections embraced by the term', *Transactions of the Royal Academy of Medicine in Ireland*, Vol. 18, No. 1 (December 1900), 68–79.

78 Langford-Symes, *RAMI*, 1900. British physician, Thomas Carleton Railton, made similar observations in 'The early symptoms of some of the infectious diseases (1890)', *LSE Selected Pamphlets*, 11–14.

79 *Registered Disease and Actual Causes of Death of all Children in the Whole of Ireland for the Ten Years ending December 31st 1896* as found in William Langford Symes, 'On the mortality of children in Ireland (1886–1896)', *Transactions of the Royal Academy of Medicine in Ireland*, Vol. 16, No. 1 (December 1898), 381–94.

annual diphtheria fatalities were nearer to 1,000 per annum. Considering that other cause of death headings, particularly, Suffocation, Laryngitis, Sore Throat and Quinsy, and Ill-defined Diseases of the Respiratory System – responsible for 4,475 deaths combined– most certainly included a significant proportion of misdiagnosed diphtheria fatalities. If misdiagnosis ran at a modest rate of 20 per cent, then it must be reasonable to suggest that diphtheria-related fatalities were more likely to be 2,000 per annum.[80]

There are two further major factors worth considering here. Firstly, the statistical record relates only to local authorities who saw fit to notify the Registrar General of outbreaks of disease in their districts, and the fatalities that ensued. As notification was not mandatory, the surviving statistical record is an unreliable representation of the country as a whole. The second issue is that figures presented for the ten years to 1896 are concerned only with children aged five years and younger. As the toll exacted by diphtheria fell heaviest on children aged between five and ten years, and that children up to the age of fifteen were regular victims of the disease, then it seems reasonable to forward the supposition that in the years prior to 1896, diphtheria had been responsible for between 2,000 and 3,000 child deaths annually. Although the surviving statistical data does not substantiate these figures, accounts of epidemic diphtheria recorded in contemporary local and national press may lend some weight to the assertion that diphtheria was far more widespread and more fatal than the statistical record suggests.

In October 1900, a 'serious epidemic of diphtheria' broke out in Kilkenny. Almost 300 cases occurred and 'a number of deaths' ensued.[81] An outbreak on this scale brought a charge of negligence against the 'so-called sanitary authorities': the incident cited as evidence to support the charge that the sanitation of Kilkenny had been 'utterly neglected' by public health authorities there.[82] This episode highlights a further reason why diphtheria remained largely absent from public health records prior to 1900: fear of recrimination. Outbreaks of infectious disease, routinely blamed on environmental factors such as defective drainage, led to afflicted towns 'getting a bad name'.[83]

In 1902, an outbreak of diphtheria 'brought to light a very serious condition of things' in Kingstown (now Dun Laoghaire). Over two weeks in September, 12 children contracted the disease and two perished. Six general

80 *Registered Disease and Actual Causes of Death of all Children in the Whole of Ireland for the Ten Years ending December 31st, 1896:* Deaths recorded for Croup (7089), Suffocation (1199), Laryngitis (742), Sore Throat and Quinsy (695), and Ill-defined Disease of the Respiratory System (1839).
81 'Local government in Kilkenny', *Irish Times*, 6 October 1900.
82 'Society gossip from the world', *Irish Times*, 3 November 1900.
83 'Health hints by a family doctor', *Irish Times*. 7 January 1905.

practitioners in the town also had cases of diphtheria under their notice, and failed to notify them. The Poor Law Guardian for Kingstown, J. J. Kenny, stressed that while he had no desire to create a scare, he cautioned 'we cannot refrain from expressing our opinion that by their absurd attitude the opponents of notification deliberately invited a dreadful visitation'.[84] Councillor W. G. Barrett of Kingstown Urban Council urged his fellow council members to adopt the Notification and Prevention of Infectious Disease Acts, but like so many other districts in Ireland, the Kingstown board members opposed the motion fearing that the town 'would lose its good name'.[85]

In County Tipperary, the clerk to the Board of Guardians and Council requested a Local Government Board (LGB) inspector to investigate an outbreak of diphtheria in the Glastrigan district of Nenagh during the summer of 1902. In September, the LGB Inspector, Dr Browne, duly reported on the outbreak, but a cohort of board members vociferously refused to accept that diphtheria existed in any of their districts. Browne stated that he would be glad to say that the south of Ireland was free from disease; however, he cautioned 'some people would like to have the doctor cloak the disease and allow it through the country. I think the members of this Board are sufficiently intelligent enough not to allow that to take place'.[86]

Browne's report illustrates the collective failure to recognize 'the true nature of the disease' – on the part of parents, general practitioners, and public representatives. No family, particularly if they were food producers, wanted their home associated with disease, and for fear of recrimination, summoned a doctor only when diphtheria had progressed to an advanced, and often-fatal stage. This undoubtedly hampered a physician's ability to treat diphtheria. However, widespread misdiagnosis and the attendant perfunctory system of notification was only partly a result of medical ignorance. Dispensary doctors sought to avoid unnecessary scrutiny, and possible recrimination, from local public health authorities to whom they relied on for patronage and remuneration.[87] While local authorities regarded notifications of croup and scarlatina as 'familiar and inevitable', notification of diphtheria implied the arrival of a new public health scourge in a district.[88]

In 1906, the Infectious Disease (Ireland) Act extended the Infectious Disease (Notification) Act of 1889 to every urban, rural, and port sanitary

---

84   *Irish Times*, 7 October 1902.
85   'Outbreak of diphtheria: Many cases in Kingstown', *Irish Times*, 29 September 1902.
86   *Nenagh News*, 20 September 1902.
87   Dorothy Porter, *Health, civilization and the state: A history of public health from ancient to modern times* (London, 1999), 135.
88   Hooker and Bashford, *Medical History*, 2002, 46.

district in Ireland.[89] Although some health districts voluntarily adopted the 1889 regulations, the 1906 measure mandated every sanitary authority to notify outbreaks of infectious disease in their districts. While the Infectious Disease (Ireland) Act added to an already impressive canon of public health legislation, implementation was haphazard: administrative structures tasked with implementing such legislation were either defective, or completely absent.[90] Nevertheless, the 1906 Act prompted a change of attitude in some districts.

In 1910, an inquest into the death of an infant from diphtheria in Dundalk Workhouse found that the child remained eight days without medical treatment.[91] The County Coroner, Dr Sellers, explained that diphtheria had been prevalent in the town for some months, and that the vast majority of diphtheria fatalities ensued because the infected children had been 'very much neglected'. Sellers charged that such a 'scandalous state of affairs [...] bordered on criminality' and undertook to hold an inquest in all future cases where he suspected diphtheria as a cause of death to direct public attention to the neglect of parents, and medical practitioners.[92] Sellers's remarks elicited some response in Dundalk: the following month saw an unprecedented 90 diphtheria cases, and 12 diphtheria fatalities, notified there.[93]

Summer 1911, saw 'an unusual number' of diphtheria cases reported in Belfast. The outbreak centred on the Antrim Road district where a number of those affected consumed milk from a dairy where a worker had full-blown diphtheria.[94] Later that year, epidemic diphtheria appeared in New Ross, County Wexford, with 50 cases admitted for treatment to the local infirmary, as the district hospital was reportedly 'full of diphtheria cases'.[95] At an emergency meeting, the urban council voted to prosecute a man who went among the population of the town while suffering from diphtheria, and had refused to go to the fever hospital.[96]

In cases where a diphtheric willingly agreed to a period of confinement, fear of the disease among healthcare workers, caused some concern. In Borrisokane, a 'bad case' of diphtheria was diagnosed and ordered to hospital, but fear of the disease was so prevalent in the town that the attending doctor

89   *Infectious Disease (Ireland) Act*, 1906.
90   Ruth Barrington, *Health, medicine, and politics in Ireland 1900–1970* (Dublin, 1987), 12–13.
91   'Diphtheria outbreak in Dundalk: Coroners strong remarks', *Irish Times*, 28 December 1910.
92   'Ireland', *British Medical Journal* (7 January 1911), 41.
93   'Recent outbreak of diphtheria in Dundalk', *Irish Times*, 2 February 1911.
94   'Ireland', *British Medical Journal* (1 July 1911), 47.
95   'An epidemic in New Ross', *British Medical Journal* (4 November 1911), 1226.
96   *British Medical Journal* (4 November 1911), 1226.

could not get anyone to accompany the child. A temporary member of staff remonstrated that it was outside her duty, then reluctantly acquiesced, and earned the gratitude of the guardians for 'her heroic act'.[97] In Castlebar, a girl developed diphtheria during a stay in the County Infirmary. The attending physician, Dr Hopkins, requisitioned an ambulance to transfer the child to the local fever hospital and recommended that a nurse accompany her. The master directed a Nurse McGee to accompany the child, but she refused, as 'it was not a portion of her duty she was appointed to discharge'. Several more nurses also refused on the same basis. The master then instructed one of the hospital maids to accompany the child, but she too declined.[98] Clearly, hospital staff at all levels were very well acquainted with diphtheria and the often-fatal consequences associated with it, implying that diphtheria was a much more common disease than the statistical record suggests.

97 *Nenagh News*, 27 January 1912.
98 *Connaught Telegraph*, 9 March 1912.

2

Diphtheria 'Arrives'

In the early twentieth century, urban centres in Britain and Ireland
experienced increased incidence of diphtheria. Dublin failed to evade
this ominous trend. In 1911, Dublin's long-standing Chief Medical
Officer, Sir Charles Cameron, conceded that 'diphtheria had been more
than usually prevalent in the city'. Cameron issued 'a serious warning' about
the dangers of the disease through local newspapers, and appealed to the
education commissioners for a temporary closure of primary schools in the
city.[1] The editor of the *Irish Times* commented: 'The terms of Sir Charles
Cameron's letter are carefully framed in order to obviate any kind of panic,
but it is clear that the authorities regard this matter with some concern'.[2]
In early February, the Dublin public health committee reported an average
increase of six new diphtheria cases per day, and by mid-February, Cameron
conceded that the disease had become 'epidemic in the city'.[3]

Prior to the introduction of the Infectious Disease (Ireland) Act, 1906,
Dublin's public health officials insisted that diphtheria had been 'a rare
disease' in the city, and diphtheria is largely absent from the statistical
record relating to this period. After 1906, diphtheria gained prominence
in Dublin. It regularly appeared in epidemic form and became endemic
throughout the city in a relatively short period. It appears that Dublin public
health authorities, under Cameron, wilfully neglected to report outbreaks
of diphtheria or to implement any intervention to combat the disease. This
grave disease, 'childhood's deadliest scourge' according to some, levied a
heavy toll on infant and child life during the nineteenth century.[4] While
it is highly unlikely that Dublin children were exempt from the ravages of
diphtheria, it is equally likely that their plight went unacknowledged by the
city's public health authorities.

---

1 'Editorial Article 4', *Irish Times*, 9 February 1911.
2 *Irish Times*, 9 February 1911.
3 'Letter from Sir Charles Cameron', *Irish Times*, 16 February 1911.
4 Hammonds, *Childhood's deadliest scourge* (Baltimore, 1999).

Lydia Carroll maintained that Cameron worked tirelessly to confront the commercial interests of Dublin property owners in a bid to protect the welfare of the powerless working poor.[5] However, when it came to outbreaks of infectious disease, Cameron regularly blamed the poor themselves for their ills. Positioning less well-off citizens as vectors, rather than victims of disease, Cameron regularly diverted blame for endemic diphtheria in the city from the sanitary authorities under his control, to the 'poorer classes' and the 'the filthy condition of the tenement houses which they occupied'. In a letter to the *Irish Times* Cameron stated:

> It is a fact that many of the tenements purlieus of the city are generally in a state far removed from cleanliness. This condition is due to personal inattention of the occupants to the most elementary elements of hygiene. They do not keep themselves, their clothing, bedding, and dwellings in a cleanly state.[6]

Cameron's strategy backfired badly. Instead of diverting blame from municipal public health services, he succeeded only in drawing the wrath of some well-respected citizens who did not shirk from levelling criticism at him, and the local authority. Florence Conan of Dalkey told the *Irish Times* that Cameron's remarks relating to tenement dwellers had 'caused anxiety in the minds of many people who are working in various ways in our poorer streets'.[7] Mrs Conan contended that the women residing in the Dublin tenements washed down their houses 'at least once a week and swept them every day'. As far as she was concerned the problem lay with the local authority and the fact that streets outside the tenements 'were not swept as often as they were in other large cities'.[8]

Municipal public health service provision also came under attack when an anonymous campaigner called on the LGB to provide anti-diphtheria antitoxin serum free of charge to all medical practitioners and dispensary medical officers as a matter of urgency, as poor patients could not afford to pay private practitioners for this lifesaving treatment. Dr Edgar Pim, Cork Street Fever Hospital, complained that Dublin's fever hospitals, tasked with carrying out 'absolutely necessary work' to prevent outbreaks of infectious disease, relied largely on voluntary conscriptions. Pim argued that municipally funded hospitals were required to treat infectious disease

---

5 Lydia Carroll, *In the fever king's preserve: Sir Charles Cameron and the Dublin slums* (Dublin, 2011).
6 'Letter from Sir Charles Cameron', *Irish Times*, 16 February 1911.
7 Florence Conan, 'Letter to the editor', *Irish Times*, 15 February 1911.
8 *Irish Times*, 15 February 1911.

effectively, but Irish hospital expenses were double their ordinary income, forcing reliance on public subscriptions.[9]

A response from 'a recent victim of what has now become epidemic', Rev. L. J. Stafford C.C., of Lower Exchange Street welcomed Cameron's letter, but wondered:

> Surely, from the head of our Public Health Department we expect more than official warning that diphtheria is rampant in our midst. It is not very consoling to be told that a plague is close upon us – it seems like reversing the first principle of hygiene, that prevention is better than cure'.[10]

In February 1911, corporation members queried Lord Mayor, Alderman Farrell, on initiatives the health committee proposed to control diphtheria. Farrell stated that 'every possible effort was being made to stamp out the disease referred to [...] money had been set aside to enable the disease to be stamped out [...] and an order had been sent out causing the public schools to be closed'.[11] Rev. Stafford, who attended the meeting, countered that apart from closing the national schools in the city, 'nothing else has been done'. Stafford challenged Cameron's assertion that 'it is almost impossible to assign a particular reason for the outbreak of diphtheria' and asserted that the statement was little more than 'a confession of ignorance that the average medical student would not like to be accused of'. In vehement condemnation, Stafford added, 'if Dublin is preserved from a plague, it will be Providence, and not the Public Health Department the people will have to thank'.[12]

Using his platform as editor at the *Irish Times* and ostensibly neutral arbiter, John Healy opined 'we cannot conceal the fact the epidemic is assuming quite serious proportions [...] and has got a firm hold on the city'.[13] Healy invited Cameron, and his staff, 'to take the citizens more fully into their confidence' as little was known as to what measures they took to curb the spread of infection. Schools closed, and the public boiled milk and water, but Healy asked if 'the resources of modern sanitary science end there?'. Healy demanded that Cameron produce 'accurate information regarding the locality of the disease'. Vague information emanating from Dublin City Hall suggested that the epidemic was prevalent on the south

---

9 Edgar Pim, 'Letter to the editor', *Irish Times*, 16 February 1911.
10 'Diphtheria in Dublin', *Irish Times*, 10 February 1911.
11 'Dublin Corporation', *Irish Times*, 14 February 1911.
12 'Disease in Dublin', *Irish Times*, 15 February 1911.
13 'Editorial article', *Irish Times*, 15 February 1911.

side of the city, which only caused alarm among residents there, and gave a false sense of security to other residential areas. Healy even demanded that Cameron publish a list of streets and suburbs reflecting the largest number of diphtheria cases, asserting that 'at such a moment we can hardly afford to respect the convenience of individuals'.[14]

Despite Cameron's focus on the tenements, and the perceived unhygienic habits of their inhabitants, the public health department subsequently revealed that the majority of diphtheria cases were furnished, not by Dublin's 'slum denizens', but by 'the middle and upper sections of the working classes residing in fairly good houses'.[15] Cameron exclaimed 'surprise' on discovering that slum and tenement dwellers 'had suffered so little from the epidemic', but declined to identify diphtheria blackspots.

During the height of the epidemic, Colonel Dopping of Blackrock urban council openly stated that 'diphtheria was rampant in Blackrock'.[16] Dopping's remark drew no immediate fire from his fellow councillors, suggesting that his assertion came as no surprise. A rebuttal subsequently came from the Blackrock medical officer, Dr J. Wallace Boyce, in the *Irish Times*.[17] At their monthly meeting, the chairman of Blackrock council, Laurence Wickham, argued that there was 'absolutely no foundation' to Dopping's claim and that 'such a serious statement would cause great hardship for every owner of property and lettor [sic] of houses in Blackrock'. Wickham suggested that medical reports 'showed no zymotic diseases, this was the case from week to week, and their health reports showed Blackrock to be the healthiest district in the United Kingdom'. Furthermore, Dr Boyce informed councillors that there was no case of diphtheria recorded, no school closed in Blackrock, and an apology should be forthcoming. The only response forthcoming from Colonel Dopping was a forthright: 'I'll stick to my guns'.[18]

Considering that the neighbouring districts of Dalkey and Booterstown experienced severe diphtheria epidemics, its absence from Blackrock was nothing short of miraculous.[19] Or, perhaps all Blackrock councillors – all but Dopping – preferred to cloak diphtheria in their district, to protect commercial interests. If so, this strategy would return to haunt them. In April 1913, rumours again surfaced at a Blackrock council meeting suggesting that the district was 'reeking with diphtheria' and that 40 fatalities had occurred in the previous weeks. The town clerk, Finlay Heron, denounced

14 *Irish Times*, 15 February 1911.
15 'Epidemic disease in Dublin', *British Medical Journal* (25 February 1911), 463.
16 'Blackrock Urban Council', *Irish Times*, 2 February 1911.
17 'The health of Blackrock', *Irish Times*, 4 February 1911.
18 'Health of the township', *Irish Times*, 16 February 1911.
19 'Dalkey school attendance committee', *Irish Times*, 21 February 1913. See also, 'Outbreak of diphtheria in Booterstown', *Irish Times*, 29 March 1913.

such rumours as 'extravagant and utterly unfounded'.[20] When it emerged
that a council member, Mr O'Hara, had lost two children to diphtheria in
the preceding days, Heron and other councillors grudgingly acknowledged
that Blackrock was in the grip of an epidemic, but insisted that it occurred
'suddenly and without warning, and came as a shock to the residents of the
district'.[21] The *British Medical Journal* blamed the Blackrock incident on 'the
consumption of contaminated milk'.[22] Although an investigation undertaken
the by the redoubtable LGB inspector, Dr Browne, failed to confirm the
'contaminated milk' theory, he did confirm that diphtheria of a severe type
was prevalent in Blackrock.[23]

Diphtheria in Cork City

From 1878, the county boroughs of Dublin, Cork, Limerick and Waterford
appointed full-time medical officers, under sanitary reforms ushered in by
the Public Health (Ireland) Act. From that year, the municipal public health
authority in Cork city compiled weekly records of the incidence of infectious
disease.[24] For the 40 years to 1918, diphtheria averaged 30 cases per year.[25]
However, in 1919, this increased to 260 notified cases, and an upward trend
continued to a peak of 588 cases in 1930.[26] The incidence of diphtheria rose
from a decennial average of 30 cases per year in 1911–20 to a decennial average
of 428 cases per year in 1921–30. The disparity might arise from a defective
method of notification prior to 1919. It may be that 'the confused administrative conditions' effected by the Great War, and concurrent Irish Revolution
hampered their efforts. If this was the case, then the extraordinary increase
in notifications recorded during the 1920s, may be more apparent than real.

It is possible that the opening and expansion of the Ford Motor Company
in Cork contributed to the increased incidence of disease in general, and
diphtheria in particular. The opening of Ford's factory in 1919 corresponds
directly with a recorded rise of over 750 per cent in the incidence of
diphtheria in the city, and the expansion of the factory in 1929 directly

20 'Diphtheria outbreak in Blackrock', *Irish Times*, 3 April 1913.
21 'Statement by sanitary authorities', *Irish Times*, 5 April 1913.
22 'Ireland', *British Medical Journal* (12 April 1913), 792.
23 'Diphtheria in Blackrock; Local Government Inspectors Report', *Irish Times*, 18 April
    1913.
24 CC&CA, CP/C/CM/PH/A/30. Weekly records of the incidence of infectious disease
    in Cork city, compiled by the municipal public health department since 1878.
25 Saunders, *Report 1931*, 20. The years 1880 and 1888 being exceptions, when the
    recorded diphtheria death rate for Cork city was 13 and 18 respectively.
26 Saunders, *Report 1931*, 19.

precedes the highest recorded rate of diphtheria in the city, which occurred during 1930. Large industrial establishments in Cork rarely employed more than 200–300 workers. By 1929, Ford employed close to 7,000 workers, and attracted 'very large numbers of employees, not only from all parts of Ireland, but also from the great industrial centres of Great Britain'.[27]

It is quite probable that a substantial proportion of the city's new population were diphtheria 'carriers'. This internal migration occurred in a city already suffering the ill effects of an acute housing shortage.[28] Dwellings for migrants were 'unprocurable, even at inflated rents' and it was not unusual 'for a Fordson worker to return home to occupy a bed that had been vacated by another employee whose shift was just commencing'.[29] In many cases four, five, and even six beds were placed in one room under conditions that made cleanliness, comfort, and proper rest impossible.[30] The rapid population increase 'taxed the resources of the city to the uttermost' and it must be reasonable to assume that opportunities for increased propagation of a highly contagious disease such as diphtheria multiplied.[31]

The wave of economic prosperity, in the wake of Ford's arrival, influenced a 20 per cent increase in the annual birth rate in the city.[32] This substantial rise increased the numbers of those most susceptible to the ravages of diphtheria. In January 1923, the resident medical officer of the Cork Fever Hospital, Dr Sutton, admitted 70 children in that month alone, 'mostly suffering from diphtheria'. Sutton attributed this to 'overcrowding and want of proper nourishment, especially for the younger children' and stated that 'underfed children in overcrowded rooms become easy victims to the ravages of the disease'.[33] His hospital management committee acknowledged that the matter was of 'deep concern to the entire community' but in light of widespread unemployment, malnourishment, and overcrowding, accepted that they could do little. During 1923, 350 diphtheria cases presented at the Fever Hospital:

27 H. A. Pelly, President of Cork Incorporated Chamber of Commerce and Shipping, 'Extension of Ford's works causes congestion in Cork', *Irish Times*, 17 February 1930. Thomas Grimes, 'Starting Ireland on the road to industry: Henry Ford in Cork' (PhD thesis, NUIG 2008). See also, Miriam Nyhan, *Are you still below? The Ford Marina Plant, Cork, 1917–1984* (Cork, 2007).
28 Cork Town Planning Association, *Cork; a civic study* (Liverpool, 1926).
29 Pelly, *Irish Times*, 17 February 1930.
30 Pelly, *Irish Times*, 17 February 1930.
31 Cork Town Planning Association, *Cork, a civic study* (1926). See also, Michael Dwyer, 'Abandoned by God and the Corporation: housing and the health of the working class in Cork City, 1912–1924', *Saothar 38, Journal of the Irish Labour History Society* (2013), 105–18.
32 The birth rate for Cork city in 1930 is recorded as being 25.4 as compared with 19.3 for the Free State as a whole and 16.3 for England & Wales. Source: Saunders, *Report of the Medical Officer of Health for the year 1930* (County Borough of Cork, 1931), 8.
33 *Cork Examiner*, 9 February 1923.

most deemed 'hopeless on admission'. The hospital treasurer, Richard Cody, lamented that the number of diphtheria admissions was an 'enormous burden for the hospital to have to shoulder' and 'hoped and prayed that some change for the better would come quickly over the state of the country'.[34]

A sharp rise in diphtheria mortality accompanied increased morbidity. For the 40 years to 1918, annual mortality rates in Cork averaged between five and seven deaths. However, in 1919–22, mortality rates in the city increased by over 1,000 per cent to an annual average of 48 deaths per year. Although an abatement of the disease from 1922–26 resulted in a much-reduced mortality rate, diphtheria mortality increased again in 1927, peaking in 1930, when 64 fatalities occurred during a period of epidemicity.[35] It is possible that diphtheria mortality may have also been skewed by defective notification and that the increase subsequent to 1918 was again more apparent than real. National diphtheria mortality rates show that pre-1918 mortality rates in Cork city were marginally higher than, but largely in line with the national rate.[36] However, from 1919 onwards, a marked divergence is discernible between a relatively constant national diphtheria mortality rate, and a significantly increased mortality rate in Cork city, a rate that corresponds directly with periods of epidemicity in the city.

During 1927, the Cork Fever Hospital committee reported that increased numbers of children from the city's congested districts presented suffering from infectious disease in general and diphtheria in particular.[37] The chairman, Sir John Scott, reported increased prevalence of scarlet fever, measles, and diphtheria, which he claimed 'had taken a stronghold in the city'.[38] Scott blamed the contagion on environmental factors, and complained to the local authority regarding the neglect of public lavatories, want of cleaning and whitewashing of lanes, and the unpleasant smell from the river.[39]

The medical officer for the Bandon dispensary, Dr D. Hennessey, affirmed that diphtheria was on the increase in Cork city and 'virtually every district in the county'. However, Hennessy looked beyond environmental factors and drew attention to the laboratory-based anti-diphtheria measures in use in America, asserting that this anti-diphtheria public health intervention had 'long since passed the experimental stage'.[40] Hennessey must

34 'Cork Fever Hospital: Prevalence of diphtheria', *Cork Examiner*, 4 January 1923.
35 Saunders, *Report 1931*, 20.
36 National rates of diphtheria mortality had rarely registered more than 1.0/1000 per population.
37 'Diphtheria in Cork', *Irish Times*, 21 July 1927, 11.
38 CC&CA, CP/C/CM/PH/A/30, Letter from Sir John Scott to Donal Carroll, Chief Superintendent Medical Officer of Health for Cork County Borough, dated 6 July 1927.
39 Letter from John Scott to Donal Carroll, 6 July 1927.
40 *Irish Times*, 21 July 1927, 11.

have made a convincing case. In July 1927, the Cork health board requested Minister for Local Government and Public Health, Richard Mulcahy, to consider making anti-diphtheria immunization compulsory.

Not all members of the health board supported Hennessey's motion. Cork city Commissioner, Philip Monahan, contested that there was no public support for immunization and because parents were already reluctant to vaccinate children against smallpox, 'it would be useless to request them to have them inoculated against diphtheria'.[41] Monahan made a valid point. In 1926, there were over 1,730 smallpox vaccination defaulters in the city.[42] Both Brunton and Kruse argued that popular resistance to smallpox vaccination in Ireland had little to do with the medical procedure itself and was motivated by anti-government sentiment in the pre-independence era.[43] Considering that the Irish Anti-Vaccination League, with such high-profile members as Eamon de Valera, George Bernard Shaw, and Francis Sheehy-Skeffington, all but disappeared post-independence, this thesis holds some water.

Despite his reservations, Commissioner Monaghan acknowledged the prevalence of diphtheria in Cork city but forcefully asserted that weak public health administration in county districts ensured that, 'it was impossible to prevent contagion spreading from areas adjoining the city, to the city itself'.[44] This was also a valid concern. Hospital accommodation in Cork rural districts was generally of 'a very limited and very unsuitable character' and medical officers often refrained from sending diphtheria patients to hospital because of a lack of hospital beds. This greatly facilitated the propagation of diphtheria and some medical officers observed that 'it was most fortunate that this virulent disease did not decimate one or two districts'.[45] Chief Medical Officer to Cork city, Dr Donal Carroll, conceded that 'it is extremely difficult to deal with infectious disease of the respiratory passage in the City as citizens are in constant intimate intercourse between [sic] the inhabitants of rural areas'.[46]

---

41 *Irish Times*, 21 July 1927, 11.
42 CC&CA. CP/C/CM/PH/A/30. Letter from Minister of Local Government and public health: No. M.53621/1926.
43 Deborah Brunton, 'The problems of Implementation: the failure and success of public vaccination against smallpox in Ireland, 1840–1873', in E. Malcolm and G. Jones, *Medicine, disease and the state in Ireland, 1650–1940*, (Cork University Press, 1999), 138–56. See also, Jutta Kruse, 'Saving Irish national infants or protecting the Irish nation? Irish anti-vaccination discourse, 1900–1930', *History Studies*, Vol. 13 (2012), 91–113.
44 *Irish Times*, 21 July 1927, 11.
45 *Cork Examiner*, 22 January 1923.
46 CC&CA, CP/C/CM/PH/A/30. Letter from Dr. D. J. Carroll, Medical Officer of Health for Cork County Borough to the Hon, Secretary and chairman, Cork Fever Hospital, July 1927.

Donal Carroll was a highly experienced medical professional. He was one of three Irish medical practitioners to train in modern public health methodologies in America under travelling fellowships supported by the Rockefeller Foundation.[47] In 1928, the main incidence of diphtheria in Ireland occurred in Cork city and county: accounting for 37 per cent and 40 per cent of cases recorded for all urban and rural areas respectively.[48] If Ireland was to adopt anti-diphtheria immunization, Cork seemed the most obvious place to start. However, within a few months of taking up his post, Carroll contracted an unspecified, and ultimately fatal illness. While incapacitated, substitute medical officers supervised public health services in the city, and the health of the city saw little or no improvement.

In May 1929, Dr Jack Saunders transferred from his post as medical officer to Cork County to succeed Donal Carroll in Cork County Borough. Saunders examined the city's health records to ascertain the position in relation to infectious disease. His investigation confirmed previously expressed fears. There was 'an undue prevalence of diphtheria' and the 'abnormal incidence' began in 1919.[49] Compared with other urban centres in Ireland and England, the rate of diphtheria morbidity and mortality rates recorded for Cork city revealed a 'disquieting situation'.[50]

Saunders secured health records from the British Ministry of Health, London County Council, and medical officers working in Birmingham, Manchester, Dublin, and Limerick.[51] Comparative analysis found that for the years 1906–18, Irish urban centres experienced a lower incidence of diphtheria than their English equivalents. During this period, Dublin, Cork, and Limerick recorded an average rate of 0.05/1000 per population, whereas London, Manchester, and Birmingham recorded an average rate of 1.08/1000: three times that of their Irish counterparts.[52]

In 1919, the incidence of diphtheria in Cork city increased sharply from 0.43/1,000 to 3.37/1,000, a rate substantially greater than that recorded for London; 2.18/1,000 for the corresponding year. London consistently

---

47 See, G. Jones, 'The Rockefeller Foundation and medical education in Ireland in the 1920s', *Irish Historical Studies*, Vol. 30, No. 120 (November 1997), 564–80; CC&CA, CP/C/CM/PH/A/30. The Cork public health records show that Carroll had ordered a copy of Graham Forbes, *Prevention against diphtheria*, in May 1927.
48 DLG&PH, *Report 1929–30*, 27–28.
49 CCCLS/352.4. J. C. Saunders, *Report of the Medical Officer of Health for the year 1931* (County Borough of Cork, 1932), 19–20.
50 Saunders, *Report for 1931*, 19–20.
51 Figures for England and Wales are available from 1911 as the central collection of notifications began that year.
52 Saunders, *Report 1931*, 21–22. The recorded incidence of diphtheria was Dublin, 0.09/1,000; Cork, 0.06/1,000; Limerick, 0.01/1,000; London 1.79/1,000; Manchester, 0.08/1,000; Birmingham, 1.39/1,000.

registered the highest average incidence of diphtheria of any city in England, though the rate of 3.37/1,000, recorded in Cork city during 1919 was, according to Graham Forbes, 'the highest rate ever recorded in any European city'. With regard to diphtheria mortality, Irish urban centres recorded far greater rates than their English counterparts. Taken in conjunction with the associated recorded rates of incidence, it seems that the majority of diphtheria cases in Ireland went undiagnosed until a fatality occurred. In 1919, diphtheria mortality in Cork city was 12.2/1,000; in Dublin, 14.4/1,000; and in Limerick, 38.4/1,000, all of which compared unfavourably with London where a rate of 8.2/1,000 prevailed. By 1930, the disparity worsened. Cork city recorded a mortality rate of 10/1,000; Dublin, 12.2/1,000; and Limerick, 18.1/1,000, compared with a greatly diminished mortality rate of 3/1,000 recorded in London.[53]

Public Health Reform in the Irish Free State

The emergence of an independent Irish Free State brought 'a gradual recovery from the confused administrative conditions' that marked the revolutionary period and subsequent Civil War. By 1923, the normal functions of public health control recovered, with renewed emphasis on medical inspections, and the methodological collection of data relating to the incidence of infectious disease.[54] The Ministry of Local Government[55] acknowledged that a 'relaxation of administrative activity' during the 'period of disturbance', ensured that the practice of reporting outbreaks of infectious disease had 'fallen into disuse'. In January 1923, the Ministry wrote to medical officers to remind them of their duties. When the practice of examining medical officer returns resumed, it became immediately apparent that a 'generalised prevalence' of diphtheria permeated the Free State.[56]

Cork city, and Newcastle West, Limerick, were adversely affected by 'a prolonged visitation of diphtheria', and public health officials in these districts maintained that defective sanitation, and poor housing, were the main agents of causation and dissemination of diphtheria during this period.[57] In Newcastle West, doctors blamed the diphtheria epidemic on a lack of adequate facilities for water supply and sewage, and the local

53 Forbes, *The Lancet*, 1927, 87.
54 Department of Local Government and Public Health, *First Report*, 1922–1925, Section II, Public Health. (Pagination unclear).
55 The Ministry of Local Government was reconstituted as the Department of Local Government and Public Health under the Ministers and Secretaries Act 1924.
56 DLG&PH, *First Report*.
57 'Rath-Luirc', *Cork Examiner*, 22 January 1923.

sanitary authority gave directions for the necessary remedial actions there. In Cork County Borough, 'an unduly high proportion' of diphtheria notifications occurred early in 1924.[58] Health Inspector, Dr John MacCormack reported that the health authorities in the city were 'quite alive' to the seriousness of the situation and were 'doing what they could' to combat it. However, MacCormack concluded that 'in view of existing circumstances of over-crowding, insanitary conditions and defective drainage, the effectual remedy consisted in an extensive housing scheme'.[59]

The duty to notify outbreaks of infectious disease rested with a network of 624 Dispensary Medical Officers (DMO) who doubled up as part-time departmental medical officers and were paid in that capacity. They submitted, or at least were obliged to submit, reports relating to outbreaks of disease in their districts. The election of a medical officer to a 'good district' could only be guaranteed by political canvassing, and remuneration for public health duties, fixed and payable by local authorities, were a constant cause of discontent and unsettlement. Dissatisfaction with the rate of remuneration and a fear of alienating political patronage induced a much-reduced sense of obligation on the part of DMOs, who routinely neglected to report outbreaks of infectious disease.[60] This suited local vested interest. It diverted unwanted scrutiny from the widespread unhygienic methods of food production, a principal factor in the propagation of infectious disease.

The reconstitution of the Ministry of Local Government as the Department of Local Government and Public Health (DLG&PH) demonstrated willingness on the part of the incumbent Cumann na nGaedheal administration to tackle national public health challenges; the Local Government Act 1925 confirmed that commitment. This act sought to reorganize local government and to centralize public health administration in each county. It placed an obligation on the minister to co-ordinate measures 'conducive to the health of the people'.[61] In addition, it placed a mandatory requirement on every County Council to appoint a full-time medical officer, responsible directly to the sanitary authorities of each county for the effective administration of the sanitary laws.[62]

These measures met with widespread opposition, and because of claimed financial difficulties, but more likely political dissent, by the end of 1925, the DLG&PH had dissolved 20 local authorities: their property, powers, and duties transferred to ministerial appointed commissioners.[63] Opposition

58 *Cork Examiner*, 22 January 1923.
59 DLG&PH, *First Report*.
60 Letter to the Editor, *Irish Independent*, 20 December 1923.
61 Department of Local Government and Public Health, *Local Government Act 1925*.
62 DLG&PH, *Local Government Act, 1925*, Section 18.
63 DLG&PH, *First Report 1922–1925*, Control of Local Authorities (pagination unclear).

parties accused the government of carrying out 'a politically motivated methodological policy of dissolution' targeting those 'who did not approve of certain work of the government of the Free State'.[64] Minister Seamus Burke responded, stating that many allegations of corruption in local government were 'untrue or exaggerated', however, he stressed that the system of filling local appointments accompanied by personal canvassing of council members was 'a cause for much dissatisfaction'.[65] The Local Authorities (Officers and Employees) Act 1926 eroded the power of local government even further by charging commissioners with controlling professional and technical local authority appointments.[66]

To ensure that newly appointed County Medical Officers (CMOs) were free from any local influence, and to establish a national service carried on merit alone, local authorities were to make appointments under the terms of the Officers and Employees Act.[67] In response, vested interests lobbied their respective health boards and councillors to block candidates of ministerial selection. Although monetary concerns were the primary reason that councils gave for avoiding employing a full-time CMO, it is possible to identify instances of localism, gender restriction, sectarianism, political patronage, and widespread anti-government sentiment, the Civil War moving from the battlefield to the council chambers.[68] Notwithstanding, this centralized control ensured that local appointments were made on merit, and not because of bribery or political influence.[69]

During 1927, departmental medical inspectors undertook a number of special investigations into outbreaks of infectious disease, as well as a series of general inspections of the sanitary administration in place in various health districts.[70] The inspections sought to place a check on the vigilance, or otherwise, of sanitary staff, and to act as 'an index of defective performance of communal functions' in relation to the adequate supply and maintenance of services relating to water supply, sewage, nuisance removal, and supervision of the food supply.[71] The DLG&PH subsequently notified local authorities

64 *Dáil Debates*, Vol. 9, 3 December 1924, folio 1964.
65 Department of Local Government and Public Health, *Second Report* (Stationery Office, Dublin), 17.
66 Eunan O'Halpin, 'Politics and the State, 1922–32', in J. R. Hill (ed.), *A new history of Ireland: VII: Ireland, 1921–84* (Oxford, 2010), 112.
67 Mary E. Daly, *The buffer state; the historical roots of the Department of the Environment* (Dublin, 1997), 131.
68 Michael Dwyer, 'Cumann na nGaedheal and the reform of public health administration in the Irish Free State', *Australasian Journal of Irish Studies*, Vol. 13 (2013), 149–63.
69 Mary E. Daly, 'Local appointments', in Mary E. Daly (ed.), *County & town*, 54.
70 DLG&PH, *Report 1929–30*, 27–28, 152–54.
71 Department of Local Government and Public Health, *Third Report* (Stationery Office, Dublin), 32–33.

of defects in connection with staff organization, or with sanitary services. However, the inspections inadvertently exposed a discrepancy in the correlation of registered deaths with the statistics of the known incidence of the 'graver epidemic diseases'. This suggested that the duty of notification continued to be 'insufficiently observed' in many districts.[72] In December 1927, a circular letter addressed to sanitary authorities stressed that the systematic notification of infectious disease was a 'fundamental element in efficient sanitary administration', and central health advised local authorities to give notice to the medical profession, and the general public, that those who defaulted in their duty of notification would be liable to penalty.[73]

The perfunctory system of notification overseen by part-time dispensary medical officers gave way to a system that mandated the submission of comprehensive weekly returns of infectious diseases, as recorded by newly appointed, independent, CMOs. However, the appointment process continued to encounter widespread, and often violent, opposition. Many counties resisted the ministerial direction to make such appointments and, by extension, remained without any semblance of a coordinated public health service, until as late as 1936. In health districts where a CMO took his position, and could discharge his duties unimpeded, it is possible to discern that they forwarded reasonably accurate, and regular, notifications to central health. The absence of a CMO in many districts, and the non-uniform rollout of appointments, suggests that the national statistical record for the period prior to 1936 is not a complete, or accurate record of infectious disease in the Free State.

Nevertheless, efforts to reform public health administration in the fledgling Free State laid the foundations for an improved system of public health service provision. Many newly appointed medical officers received training in contemporary public health methodologies in America, and all appointees held a Diploma in Public Health in addition to medical degrees. The timing of these appointments proved crucial in the drive to control diphtheria in the Free State, as they coincided with the emergence of international public health interventions that successfully dislodged traditional sanitarian approaches to disease control in favour of bacteriological and immunological interventions. However, as facilities to manufacture anti-diphtheria serums were not available in Ireland, Irish public health doctors would have to rely on work undertaken in foreign laboratories to procure a steady supply of a safe and efficient prophylactic.

72 DLG&PH, *Third Report*, 33.
73 'Notification of disease: Tightening up the law in Free State', *Irish Times*, 8 December 1927.

The Development of Antitoxin
as an Anti-diphtheria Prophylactic

Until the late nineteenth century, physicians' understanding of disease causation included explanations that blamed the occurrence on agents of the occult, miasma, and an association with damp and cold weather.[74] Louis Pasteur's germ theory paved the way for a biological explanation of disease, and improved methods of diagnosis, treatment, and prevention owe much to the work of Robert Koch.[75] In 1883, German microbiologist, Edwin Klebs, identified the bacterium *Corynebacterium diphtheria* in pseudo membranes removed from diphtheria patients and a year later his compatriot, and one of Koch's assistants, Friedrich Loeffler, succeeded in cultivating it. Loeffler successfully isolated the specific diphtheria organism from throat swabs taken from clinically confirmed diphtheria cases by growing the bacterium on a special type of medium, which still bears his name. When Loeffler injected the diphtheria bacillus into animals, he found that characteristic diphtheria membranes and other lesions appeared, closely resembling the pseudo membrane found at autopsy in human cases of diphtheria. Loeffler suggested, but could not definitively prove that the diphtheria bacillus caused death by 'elaborating a powerful, extracellular poison or toxin'.[76]

Many experiments with the Klebs-Loeffler bacillus during the 1880s and 1890s succeeded in producing a toxin and although it was not very potent or pure, this work served as a significant building block for Émile Roux and Alexander Yersin in France, and Emil Behring and Shibasaburo Kitasato in Germany, who first introduced diphtheria 'antitoxin' in 1890. In preliminary experiments Carl Fraenkel, a colleague of Behring and Kitasato at the Institute of Infectious Disease, Berlin, discovered that if he injected a toxic substance extracted from diphtheria cultures into animals in sub-lethal doses, the animal produced a specific immunity against the diphtheria bacillus and its toxic product.[77]

Both Behring and Fraenkel independently observed that serum produced from animals who survived sub-lethal doses of diphtheria bacillus acquired a new property: 'it now contained something which enabled it to prevent the harmful effect of many lethal doses of the diphtheria bacilli and its toxin'.[78]

---

74 Joseph Robins, *The miasma: Epidemic and panic in nineteenth-century Ireland* (Dublin, 1995).

75 Roy Porter, *The greatest benefit to mankind: a medical history of humanity from antiquity to the present* (London, 1997), 438–39.

76 Parish, *Immunization*, 119.

77 Derek S. Linton, *Emil von Behring: Infectious disease, immunology, serum therapy* (Philadelphia, 2005).

78 Parish, *Immunization*, 120–21.

The German work created a worldwide sensation. The serum was first clinically trialled in 1891 and diphtheria antitoxin was first used successfully on a young girl in a Berlin clinic that same year.[79] Following some further clinical successes, Meister, Lucius and Bruning began commercial production of Behring's antitoxin serum, and its rollout into Berlin hospitals in 1894 induced a rapid plunge in diphtheria mortality there.[80]

In Paris, Roux, and Yersin, built on the success of their German counterparts and utilized horses to mass produce antitoxin. Roux's horse serum successfully treated 300 cases at the Hospital des Enfants Malades, Paris, reducing diphtheria mortality there from 52 to 25 per cent. In September 1894, at the International Congress of Hygiene and Demography, Budapest, the results of Roux's new treatment 'rapidly excited world-wide interest' and was soon established in many countries.[81]

While on a visit to Paris, the British surgeon and pioneer of antiseptic surgery, Sir Joseph Lister obtained Roux's serum and brought it to Edward Wilberforce Goodall at the Eastern Hospital, Homerton, London, where in the summer of 1894, the first British diphtheria cases received antitoxin. In the same year, Marc Armand Ruffer, a former pupil of Pasteur, prepared antitoxin at the British Institute of Preventative Medicine, London. With the help of Charles Scott Sherrington of the veterinary charity, the Browne Institute, they produced the first British-made anti-diphtheria serum. On 15 October 1894, Sherrington administered the antigen to a seven-year-old boy suffering from the advanced stages of diphtheria. The boy, George Sturgeon, recovered and use of the serum extended to hospital practice in London later that year.

The utilization of antitoxin serum as a passive immunizing agent gained widespread support among clinicians, many of whom began to consider the possibility of using the serum in a preventive capacity. It was one thing to administer an antigen to a sick child, whose chances of surviving diphtheria could be as low as one in four, but active immunization meant injecting healthy children with a toxic substance. Early pioneers, such as Dziergowski in 1903, demonstrated (using himself as a test subject) that the introduction of minute and increasing doses of toxin could induce immunity in human subjects. Dziergowski's method was protracted, painful, potentially lethal, and did not find a wide audience.[82] In 1907, American epidemiologist,

---

79 Porter, *The greatest benefit to mankind*, 438–39.
80 Frederick Crum, *Am J Public Health* (1917), 445. See also, Roy Porter (London, 1997), 438–39.
81 Parish, *Immunization*, 122.
82 J. G. Fitzgerald, 'Diphtheria toxoid as an immunizing agent', *Journal of the Canadian Medical Association*, Vol. 17, No. 5, (May 1927); 524–29. See also, George Rosen, *A history of public health* (Baltimore, 2003), 312–13.

Theobald Smith, experimented with toxin and antitoxin to create a 'neutral mixture', to vaccinate against diphtheria. His successful experiments using guinea pigs led Smith to suggest that his method could be trialled in human subjects, but he did not follow up on this.[83] However in 1913, Emile von Behring, successfully demonstrated that the injection of a neutral toxin-antitoxin mixture into a human subject produced a relatively safe, rapid, and lasting immunity against diphtheria.[84]

In the same year, Hungarian paediatrician, Bela Schick, discovered that a small dose of diphtheria toxin injected into the skin near the wrist produced a red spot after a day or two: indicating that the subject had no natural immunity to diphtheria. The Schick test was a simple and effective means of differentiating between persons who were Schick positive (susceptible to diphtheria) and Schick negative (immune to diphtheria). The Schick test effectively limited the use of toxin-antitoxin to those without natural immunity against diphtheria only, sparing the naturally immune the necessity of treatment.[85] The Schick test, and subsequent standardization of toxin-antitoxin, paved the way for the practical application of active immunization against diphtheria on a large scale, and William Park and Abraham Zingher undertook the first scheme of its type in New York children's institutions in 1913.[86]

Park, a nose and throat specialist in Manhattan, headed the New York diphtheria diagnostic laboratory from 1894, and subsequently became director of the research laboratories there. In collaboration with Anna Williams,[87] Park discovered the 'Park Williams 8' strain of *C. diphtheria*, and formulated the first diphtheria antitoxin produced outside a European laboratory. Prior to the introduction of active immunization, the death rate from diphtheria in New York stood at 18.8/100,000, representing 2,733 diphtheria fatalities per year. However, the introduction of active immunization in New York affected an immediate and substantial decrease in diphtheria mortality.[88] Park's ground-breaking intervention inspired many more North American health

83 Fitzgerald, *JCMA*, 1927, 525.
84 Parish, *Immunization*, 143.
85 William Park and Abraham Zingher, 'Diphtheria immunity-natural, active and passive. Its determination by the Schick Test', *American Journal of Public Health*, Vol. VI, No. 5 (May 1916), 431.
86 Park and Zingher, 'The control of diphtheria', *American Journal of Public Health*, Vol. 13, No. 1 (January 1923), 26. For an in-depth analysis of Parks interventions see Evelynn Hammonds, *Childhood's deadliest scourge: The campaign to control diphtheria in New York City, 1880–1930* (Baltimore, 1999).
87 For more on Anna Williams (1863–1954) see King-Thom Chung, *Women pioneers of medical research: Biographies of twenty-five outstanding scientists* (North Carolina, 2010) 48–51.
88 William C. Bosanquet and John Eyre, *Serums, vaccines and toxins in treatment and diagnosis* (London, 1909).

authorities to adopt active immunization, in their districts and by 1918, over 250,000 children had been treated in New York alone, 179,000 in Chicago, and 58,000 in Boston.[89] In continental Europe, mainly due to the persistent advocacy of a French veterinarian, Gaston Ramon, active immunization garnered support in France, Belgium, and Holland.[90]

The American intervention found some advocates among public health officials in Britain. In 1925, Dr George Buchan, president of the Society of Medical Officers of Health in London, lamented that 'the methods in vogue for the prevention of diphtheria had not met with success'.[91] Buchan informed his membership that schemes utilizing the Schick test followed by active immunization 'had been demonstrated by reliable scientific observers and clinical workers as a means by which the prevalence of diphtheria could be reduced' and he urged health departments in England to offer such schemes to the public.[92] In May 1927, Graham Forbes published a comprehensive survey of methods employed against diphtheria and in particular the use of the Schick Test and antitoxin treatment, which he hailed as 'one of the most notable advances in the sphere of preventive medicine'.[93] The British Medical Research Council agreed, and pointing to existing evidence, expressed their hope that 'diphtheria and its often-fatal consequences may now fairly be called avoidable'.[94]

In 1927, spokesman for the British health ministry, Sydney Copeman, assured members of the Society of Medical Officers of Health that the Ministry of Health fully appreciated 'the value of Schick testing combined with active immunization to combat diphtheria' and advised that more direct propaganda advocating the procedure should be conveyed to the public.[95] However, some attendees, including the influential press baron and President of the London Free Hospital, Lord George Riddell, questioned the desirability or necessity of such an intervention. In the same year, and in reaction to the publication of Forbes report, the London public health committee undertook to monitor the results of the new methods of prevention. However,

89 'Mortality from diphtheria decreasing', *American Journal of Public Health*, Vol. 16, No. 6 (June 1926), 621. See also: Saunders, *Report 1931*, 25. For an in-depth report on the roll out of anti-diphtheria immunization in America, see Selwyn D. Collins, 'History and frequency of diphtheria immunizations and cases in 9,000 families', *Public Health Reports* (1896–1970), Vol. 51, No. 51 (18 December 1936), 1736–73.
90 Parish, *Vaccines*, 93.
91 G. F. Buchan, 'Society of Medical Officers of Health', *British Medical Journal* (24 October 1925), 751.
92 Buchan, *British Medical Journal* (1925), 752.
93 'Diphtheria', *Irish Times*, 18 May 1927.
94 *Irish Times*, 18 May 1927.
95 'Campaign against diphtheria; Health Ministry and the Schick method', *The Times*, 22 January 1927, 9.

the committee subsequently decided not to recommend the introduction of active immunization for schoolchildren on the rationale that cessation of epidemics was most likely due to natural immunization through exposure to the disease, due to 'the salting of the community'.[96]

Others were more aggressive in voicing their opposition. In June 1928, Labour Councillor, Richard Lundy of Manchester City Council exclaimed:

> First vaccination, then inoculation, now immunization from diphtheria. If things develop as they are going, when a child reaches the age of 15 he will be leaving school like a complete postage stamp-perforated from head to foot. We are being asked to allow elementary schools to be used purely as experimental centres.[97]

Some London medical officers saw a more pressing need for active immunization, and the local medical officer Cecil Hutt pioneered anti-diphtheria immunization schemes in the Borough of Holborn.[98] Although London County Council sought to allay anxiety 'in the desire to tone down the degree of blackness' in London's diphtheria record, by the end of 1927 immunization schemes were inaugurated in just five of the 29 London boroughs.[99] Where schemes were adopted they were said to have been initiated by 'enthusiasts', and a government sponsored immunization scheme remained absent in Britain until wartime conditions forced their introduction during 1941.[100]

In the Irish Free State, health authorities acknowledged that the method by which diphtheria is spread 'is now probably understood better than any other infection', and with reference to the New York intervention, central health showed appreciation of the role that active immunization with antitoxin had played in reducing diphtheria mortality there.[101] This demonstrates a profound shift in the department's understanding, and attitude to communicable disease in general, and to diphtheria in particular. Previous health reports acknowledged the prevalence of diphtheria and decried the associated levels of excess child mortality, however, the contemporary recommended and accepted public health response to diphtheria was hitherto framed in a decidedly sanitarian mindset, with an emphasis on segregation and disinfection. The DLG&PH's *Third Report*, which coincided with the publication of, and was most likely influenced and informed by Graham Forbes's *The Prevention of Diphtheria*, demonstrated

96 'War on diphtheria', *Irish Times*, 29 November 1927.
97 'The treatment of diphtheria', *Irish Times*, 7 June 1928.
98 'Campaign against diphtheria', *The Times*, 22 January 1927, 9.
99 'Diphtheria in London', *Lancet*, 23 July 1927, 203.
100 Parish, *Vaccines*, 91–93.
101 DLG&PH, *Third Report, 1925–28*, 'Diphtheria', 34.

a clear knowledge of the aetiology, and method of propagation of diphtheria. More importantly, it acknowledged that the application of antitoxin as a preventive, as well as a curative measure, had been hugely successful in reducing diphtheria related mortality in New York. This is significant, as it demonstrates the willingness of the Cumann na nGaedheal administration to instigate a complete revision of long held views related to disease causation and propagation, and it demonstrates willingness to translate advances in medical science into services designed to prevent ill health, and premature death.

Diphtheria antitoxin was available in the Free State as a curative measure; however, its availability was largely restricted to fee-paying patients, and to confirmed cases of clinical diphtheria only. In 1927, central health made a clear commitment to utilize antitoxin not only to treat diphtheria, but also to 'control and effectively wipe-out this dreaded disease of childhood'.[102] The department encouraged newly appointed medical officers to adopt the Schick test and toxin-antitoxin immunization treatment in their respective districts and promoted this 'safe and simple method' as the best way of protecting against diphtheria. Previous negative experience with compulsory smallpox vaccination[103] led central health to deem it 'inadvisable' to make 'too strenuous efforts' to persuade parents to have to present children for immunization. However, in districts where the disease threatened to become epidemic they advised that 'parents should be informed that active immunization provided a safe, practicable and effective method of prevention'.[104] As James Colgrove observed of the introduction of mass childhood immunization in New York, the model for introducing anti-diphtheria immunization in Ireland also 'located the source of the disease within the individual rather than the environment, and saw persuasion rather than compulsion as the most appropriate and powerful tool for effecting change'.[105]

102 DLG&PH, *Third Report*, 34–36.
103 See Deborah Brunton, 'The problems of implementation: the failure and success of public vaccination against smallpox in Ireland, 1840–1873', in Jones and Malcolm, *Medicine, disease and the state in Ireland*, 138–57. Also, Jutta Kruse, 'Saving Irish national infants or protecting the infant nation? Irish anti-vaccination discourse, 1900–1930', *History Studies*, Vol. 13 (2012), 91–113. For the English context see Dorothy Porter and Roy Porter 'The politics of prevention: Anti-vaccinationism and public health in nineteenth century England', *Medical History*, Vol. 32, No. 3 (July 1998), 231–52.
104 DLG&PH, *Third Report*, 35.
105 James Colgrove, *State of immunity: The politics of vaccination in twentieth-century America* (California, 2006), 93.

3

Anti-diphtheria Immunization
in the Irish Free State

In November 1928, a scheme for 'the eradication of diphtheria' launched
in the Urban District of Dundalk and the adjacent rural area of County
Louth under the supervision of newly appointed county medical officer,
Dr John Musgrave. Musgrave estimated that 3,500 children aged six months
to six years would require immunization treatment to guarantee a successful
scheme. Although Musgrave, alluded to 'loose talk calculated to undermine
public confidence in the effectiveness of the work',[1] by the end of 1928, 1,500
children received the full course of treatment with no ill effects.[2] Louth
traditionally supplied the second largest contingent of urban diphtheria cases
after Cork city; by 1929 Musgrave's intervention radically altered Dundalk's
unenviable position on that league table. During 1928, Louth's urban centres,
Drogheda and Dundalk, registered five, and 43 diphtheria cases respectively.
During 1929, Drogheda recorded an increase of over 800 per cent with 41
notified cases, while Dundalk recorded a decrease of over 50 per cent with
just 20 notifications.[3]

Satisfied with the results of Musgrave's work, in April 1929, the
DLG&PH introduced the Public Health (Infectious Diseases) Regulations.
This legislation empowered sanitary authorities and county medical officers
to 'organise arrangements for testing susceptibility to diphtheria infection
and for the administration of protective agents'.[4] During 1929, immunization schemes sprang into operation in selected areas where diphtheria was
prevalent, and in health districts under the supervision of a full-time medical
officer. Diphtheria scourged Kildare, Wexford, and Tipperary that year, yet

---

1 'Immunization of Dundalk children', *Irish Times*, 11 February 1929.
2 Department of Local Government and Public Health, *Fourth Report 1928–29*
(Stationery Office, Dublin), 40.
3 Department of Local Government and Public Health, *Report 1929–30*, 28.
4 The Public Health (Infectious Disease) Regulations, 1929, Amendment No.4.

health boards in these counties remained embroiled in protracted disputes with central health over the cost of employing full-time medical officers. As a result, children residing there continued to suffer the ill effects, and often-fatal consequences associated with diphtheria.

Reporting on the prevalence of diphtheria in his district, departmental health inspector, Robert McDonnell, observed 'a very marked increase on former years'. During 1929, 322 cases occurred, a 360 per cent increase on the 70 cases recorded the previous year.[5] McDonnell opined that the substantial increase in diphtheria notifications was more apparent than real and blamed the improved system of notification, which 'the advent of the Medical Officers of Health have brought about'. He acknowledged that diphtheria had been endemic in the Dundalk district for some years, and that Musgrave's intervention influenced a marked decrease in incidence there. He conceded that the much-diminished incidence of diphtheria in Dundalk 'stood anomalously against the general trend of increased incidence of diphtheria' in every other district under his charge, but lamented that the value of immunization as a preventive measure 'does not appear to be fully appreciated by the public'.[6]

Health Inspector Winslow Sterling-Berry reported that diphtheria was also on the increase in every district under his charge, that the disease was general throughout his area, and that 336 cases occurred during 1929. Sterling-Berry noted that an anti-diphtheria immunization scheme commenced in Tullamore, County Offaly, during the year and he hoped that this would influence an amelioration of the disease there.[7] Inspector, John MacCormack, observed that the only notifiable disease in his district was diphtheria, which 'assumed epidemic proportions' in Cork city, Cork rural district, and Clonmel'.[8] During 1929, diphtheria occurred in 60 health districts under MacCormack's control: 18 urban, and 42 rural districts. Diphtheria was also prevalent in the three county boroughs encompassed by MacCormack's southern district, with 368 cases reported in Cork city, 28 cases in Limerick city, and six cases in Waterford city. Of the 462 cases

5 R. P. McDonnell was the departmental health inspector for the Borough of Dublin, Cavan, Donegal, Dunlin County, Leitrim, Longford, Louth, Meath, Monaghan, and Westmeath.

6 R. Percy McDonnell, 'Medical Inspector, on the public health of the district under his charge', in DLG&PH, *Report 1929–30*, 152.

7 Winslow Sterling-Berry, Medical Inspector, 'On the public health of the district under his charge', *Report 1929–30*, 153–54. Sterling-Berry was the DLG&PH health inspector in charge of Galway, Mayo, Sligo, Roscommon, Offaly, Kildare, Carlow, Wicklow, and Wexford.

8 John J. MacCormack, Medical Inspector, 'On the public health of the district under his charge', *Report 1929–30*, 154–64. MacCormack was the DLG&PH health inspector for Munster, Kilkenny, and Laois.

notified in southern rural districts, 371 cases, or 80 per cent occurred in County Cork.[9]

MacCormack's report confirms that diphtheria remained entrenched in Cork city and its immediate environs. For the year ending 31 March 1930, increased incidence occurred in both urban and rural areas of the county, up by 299 cases on the previous year. Cork County alone accounted for 35 per cent of all diphtheria notifications in the Free State.[10] During 1929, Dr Jack Saunders inaugurated an immunization scheme in Cork city and his counterpart Dr Robert Condy mirrored this in Cork county. By March 1930, almost 2,700 children received treatment in city schools or, at weekly immunization sessions at the municipal public health clinic at Parnell Place. In Cork county, Condy's schemes operated chiefly in the Cork rural district, and in the urban districts of Passage West, and Youghal. Fermoy councillors gave an undertaking to implement a scheme, but subsequently withdrew due to a dispute relating to Condy's travelling expenses. Inspector MacCormack, was reticent to declare any marked improvement in districts operating immunization schemes, but asserted that 'good results are confidently anticipated in the current year when the total numbers immunised will be sufficiently great to show an appreciable effect'.[11]

During 1930, increased virulence of diphtheria occurred throughout the Free State. Medical officers notified 2,992 cases and 386 fatalities. Cork again experienced the vilest visitation, registering 238 urban and 563 rural cases, accounting for 25 per cent of all non-urban cases. Tipperary South recorded the second highest incidence with 191 notified cases, the majority of which related to an epidemic in Clonmel.[12] An investigation into the continued spread of the disease in Clonmel found that the district hospital routinely discharged diphtheria patients before they fully recovered. Best practice dictated that three negative throat swabs should be obtained from patients before discharge, but in Clonmel the practice had been abandoned, and discharged children returned to school while still highly infective.[13]

In 1930, Sterling-Berry noted a continued upward trend in notifications throughout his western district. During the year, 498 cases occurred, up from 336 cases in the preceding year, the situation exacerbated by a severe epidemic in Galway Urban District, contributing 48 cases. In the Eastern inspection district, Robert McDonnell noted a similar trend. Here, 348 cases occurred, an increase of 26 on the previous year. Although the immunization scheme

9 MacCormack, DLG&PH *Report 1929–30*, 154–64.
10 DLG&PH, *Report 1929–30*, 27–28.
11 MacCormack, DLG&PH *Report 1929–30*, 154–64.
12 Department of Local Government and Public Health, *Report 1930–31* (Stationery Office, Dublin), 48–49.
13 MacCormack, DLG&PH, *Report 1930–31*, 197.

undertaken in Dundalk significantly reduced the incidence of diphtheria there, the neighbouring district, Drogheda, witnessed 'a remarkable increase' in incidence, registering 63 cases when the previous highest number reported there had not exceeded 13.[14]

By the end of 1930 immunization schemes operated, to varying degrees, in Cork and Dublin county boroughs, Dundalk, Bray, New Ross, Passage West, Tullamore, and throughout the Cork county health district.[15] Although diphtheria morbidity continued its upward trend in rural areas, the combined efforts of these disparate schemes succeeded in effecting the first recorded national decline in diphtheria morbidity and mortality over the previous five years. During 1931, national figures relating to diphtheria show that morbidity and mortality rates decreased by 18 per cent. The improvement, mostly confined to urban areas, reflected the extraordinary 55 per cent decrease in incidence recorded in Cork city and the balance related to improved figures from Clonmel and Drogheda.[16] Similarly, reduced diphtheria mortality reflected the striking reduction in the number of diphtheria related deaths in Cork city, which fell from 76 fatalities in 1930 to 27 in 1931, accounting for over 70 per cent of the reduction in national diphtheria mortality figures recorded for the year.[17]

The extraordinary results attendant on Jack Saunders's intervention influenced Cork health authorities to extend their anti-diphtheria immunization services and to incorporate child immunization as a routine part of public health administration in the city. Furthermore, the success of the Cork scheme inspired many more medical officers to inaugurate or expand immunization services in their districts. Dublin health authorities ran immunization clinics three times each week, in three city-centre venues, and by the end of 1931, 1,573 children presented for treatment. Immunization services in Dublin were coordinated with the assistance of the Maternity and Child Welfare Scheme and maintained a focus on pre-school children exclusively. Despite these efforts, diphtheria remained endemic in Dublin, and central health directed chief medical officer, Dr Matt Russell, to reorganize his immunization schemes to replicate those operated by Jack Saunders in Cork city.[18]

In Cork county, Robert Condy oversaw an extension of anti-diphtheria immunization schemes and by the end of 1931 over 5,500 children received treatment. In Passage West, a district previously disproportionally affected

14 McDonnell, DLG&PH, *Report 1930–31*, 191.
15 DLG&PH, *Report 1930–31*, 48–49, and 193.
16 Department of Local Government and Public Health, *Report 1931–32* (Stationery Office, Dublin), 43–44.
17 DLG&PH, *Report 1931–32*, 43–44.
18 DLG&PH, *Report 1931–32*, 44.

by diphtheria, an immunization scheme significantly reduced diphtheria notifications, which fell from 61 cases in 1929, to 22 in 1930, and with just two cases occurring during 1931. Similarly, in Cavan, epidemic diphtheria was a common occurrence in the Arva portion of Cavan rural district. During 1931, 'some hundreds of children' were immunized by the local medical officer, and by the end of the year, only one case occurred in the area, and this 'occurred in a child who had not being immunised'.[19] Immunization of susceptible children continued at public health clinics in New Ross, Tullamore, and Galway. By the end of 1931, almost 4,000 children received full immunization treatment in these districts and 'no child who received three injections contracted the disease'.[20]

Despite these successes, diphtheria continued to be prevalent in the Free State, particularly in rural districts. In the Eastern District, incidence increased from 70 cases in 1929, to 322 cases in 1930, and to 375 cases in 1931. In the Western District, a similar trend saw incidence increase from 336 cases in 1929, to 498 cases in 1930, and to 544 cases in 1931. In the Southern District, diphtheria remained endemic in several districts, notably Clonmel, Ennis Urban District, Killmallack Rural District, Rathkeale Rural District, and Listowel Rural District. During 1931, diphtheria appeared in 16 urban, and 60 rural districts, compared with 15 urban, and 49 rural districts in the previous year. Health Inspector Robert McDonnell again asserted that 'the improved machinery' reporting diphtheria cases 'must account for many cases being notified which formerly nothing would have been heard'.[21] McDonnell's assertion may be somewhat reductionist, but there is little doubt that the continued rollout of full-time county medical officers resulted in increased notifications. Although increased notifications may have been, as McDonnell asserted, 'more apparent than real', the improved method of notification made it patently clear that the endemic nature of diphtheria in the Free State was very real indeed.

In the Southern District, Inspector MacCormack was convinced that diphtheria was actually becoming more prevalent in rural areas and suggested that this extension was 'purely and simply the result of improved travel facilities'.[22] According to MacCormack, 'the ubiquitous bus was not an unmixed blessing' and while public transport brought remote areas within easy reach of towns and cities it also brought rural dwellers into contact with 'every manner of infection [...] and some are bound to succumb and carry back with them the germs of an infectious fever such as diphtheria'.

19 McDonnell, *Report 1931–32*, 193.
20 W. S. Sterling-Berry, *Report 1931–32*, 194–96.
21 McDonnell, *Report 1931–32*, 193.
22 MacCormack, *Report 1931–32*, 197–98.

MacCormack's anti-urban sentiments may hold a modicum of truth. However, it is more likely that infectious disease in general migrated from rural to urban centres through the conduit of adulterated meat and milk products.[23] The Clean Milk Campaign, introduced in 1926, did little to stem the supply of 'dirty Irish milk' which took a heavy toll on the health and life expectancy of infants in urban centres well into the 1950s.[24] Similarly, high-profile disputes, such as the 1930 standoff between the Dublin Public Health Department and the owners of Donnelly's Bacon Factory, served to highlight how food producers regularly and knowingly allowed adulterated meat products to enter the food chain.[25]

In 1932, and in common with most other Northern European countries, diphtheria increased in the Free State. Notifications rose substantially to 2,938, an increase of 9 per cent on the previous year, and were entirely attributable to acute outbreaks of the disease in inner city areas of Limerick, and in Dublin. In 1932 notifications in Limerick city alone increased by 274, and notifications in Dublin city increased by 224. Conversely, Cork city bucked this trend and registered a reduction of 192 notifications. While rural and smaller urban areas also registered reduced notifications, acute outbreaks occurred in the urban districts of Galway, Carlow, Monaghan, Dundalk, Tullamore, and Bray, and in the county health districts of Cork, Bandon, Mallow, Galway, Tuam, Listowel, Rathkeale, and Limerick.[26] In Galway Urban District, returns were swelled by 'multiple outbreaks of diphtheria' in Galway Central Hospital, the cause of which were attributed to undetected diphtheria carriers who infected at least 22 patients before they were discovered.[27]

Increased mortality again accompanied increased morbidity and this was evident in both urban and rural districts. National figures for 1932 show that 383 people died of diphtheria: 176 in urban and 207 in rural districts. Diphtheria fatalities in Limerick city rose dramatically from eight, to 22, and fatalities in Waterford city doubled from two to four. However, the largest number of fatal cases occurred in Dublin city, which registered 82 fatalities, an increase of ten on the previous year. In county districts, Galway experienced the highest number of fatalities, increasing from 16 to 39.

23 MacCormack's anti-urban sentiments echo those raised by Eoin Devereux, 'Saving rural Ireland: Muintir na Tire and its anti-urbanism, 1931–1958', *The Canadian Journal of Irish Studies*, Vol. 17, No. 2 (Dec. 1991), 23–30.

24 Lindsey Earner-Byrne, *Mother and child: Maternity and child welfare in Dublin, 1922–60*, (Manchester University Press, 2013).

25 *Irish Times*, 9 January 1930.

26 Department of Local Government and Public Health, *Report 1932–33* (Stationery Office, Dublin), 42.

27 DLG&PH, *Report 1932–33*, 43.

Substantial increases also occurred in rural districts in Cork, Kerry, Louth, Kilkenny, and Westmeath.[28] These deplorable figures were again countered by a sustained decrease in Cork city, where the bill of diphtheria mortality reduced by ten.

By the end of 1932, the direct correlation between levels of diphtheria in a district, and the efficiency, or otherwise, of the anti-diphtheria immunization schemes operating in a district was becoming increasingly clear to public health authorities. The experience of those involved in the longest running scheme, that being Musgrave's intervention in Dundalk, was testament to this. In Dundalk urban and rural districts, where diphtheria was once endemic, just 12 cases and two fatalities occurred during 1931. This diminution in incidence was a direct result of the intensive immunization campaign undertaken by Musgrave during 1928 and 1929. However, the success of the Dundalk campaign elicited over-confidence in the prolonged durability of active immunization among one section of Dundalk parents, and another section who remained unconvinced by the benefits of immunization remained reticent to submit their children for treatment. This combination resulted in much-diminished attendances at Musgrave's clinic and poor numbers during 1930 forced a suspension of the Dundalk campaign.[29]

The resultant natural increase in unimmunized, and thereby susceptible children during the intervening period, facilitated a recrudescence of diphtheria in Dundalk. During 1932, 49 cases, and nine case fatalities occurred in Dundalk town alone, compared with 60 cases and 13 case fatalities for County Louth as a whole. Musgrave claimed that the fall in attendance was attributable to an amount of 'lay propaganda against immunization' in the district, which he asserted was not driven by any motives beyond 'loose thinking, loose talk, and idle gossip'.[30] In June 1932, a visitation of diphtheria in epidemic form proved a timely reminder of the dangers associated with the disease. Over 500 children presented for treatment in that month alone. Many parents and medical practitioners in Louth harboured doubts about active immunization, or concerns relating to the safety of the process, but few could dispute the statistics. While 380 diphtheria cases occurred in Dundalk during the period 1928–32, only one had received immunization treatment.[31] Of the remaining 379 cases, none had received immunization treatment.

In Cork County, increased public confidence facilitated an extension of Robert Condy's immunization services into districts where diphtheria

28 DLG&PH, *Report 1932–33*, 43.
29 DLG&PH, *Report 1932–33*, 43.
30 'Fighting diphtheria', *Irish Times*, 7 January 1931.
31 DLG&PH, *Report 1932–33*, 43.

remained prevalent. During 1932, 2,801 children presented for treatment, bringing the total number treated over the previous four years to 8,305. Over the corresponding period, a sharp reduction in diphtheria notifications ensued. For the Cork Rural District as a whole, notifications fell from 216 in 1929 to just 45 during 1932. The most striking reduction occurred in the previously most adversely affected area of Cork County, Passage West. Here, notifications fell from 61 in 1929, to a single diphtheria notification during 1932. In sharp contrast, children residing in the same county, whose health boards failed to introduce active immunization, continued to suffer the ill effects of diphtheria. For instance, Mallow Rural District recorded 44 diphtheria notifications and 15 fatalities, giving a case mortality rate of 33 per cent: double the rate of the south Cork district in general. Similarly, in Bandon, 43 diphtheria cases resulted in seven fatalities, and a relatively high case mortality rate of 16.2 per cent.[32]

For the twelve years to 1930, diphtheria 'ravaged' Cork city: appearing regularly, and frequently in epidemic form. While some 6,687 cases notified in this period it is likely that thousands more went undiagnosed, were misdiagnosed, and went un-notified. An intensive immunization campaign between June 1929 and December 1932 facilitated the full treatment of almost 7,000 children, and 1,149 more received one, or two, injections over the corresponding period. This intervention effected an 85 per cent reduction in the incidence of diphtheria in the city, but failed to avert 17 diphtheria fatalities there during 1932. Ten of the seventeen deaths were children whose parents refused to have them immunized. The DLG&PH lamented: 'The preventable loss thus sustained is rendered the more poignant by the fact that of the 6,878 children who were immunised, not a single one died'.[33]

Diphtheria continued in epidemic form in several southern districts during 1932, most notably in Killaloe, Bandon, Millstreet, Buttevant, Caherciveen, Lixnaw, Abbeyleix, and Rathkeale. Although acute outbreaks occurred, to a large degree, in districts where schemes were perfunctory or non-existent, some of the blame related to confusion amongst local doctors regarding diphtheria. A number of predisposing causes such as 'bad drainage', 'too close proximity of manure heaps', and 'drinking bad water' were frequently cited in medical reports to explain the origin of the disease.[34]

It seems clear that some medics did not fully grasp the concept of the carrier menace in diphtheria infection or that it was on this understanding that protective and preventive measures against the spread of diphtheria should be organized. It seems equally clear, that in many districts, reliance on

32 DLG&PH, *Report 1932–33*, 43.
33 DLG&PH, *Report 1932–33*, 44.
34 DLG&PH, *Report 1932–33*, 205.

bacteriological examination before discharge from hospital, and arrangements for outside observation and exclusion from school of afflicted children, took second place behind a reliance on traditional sanitarian attitudes to controlling disease. In districts where health authorities remained married to Victorian concepts of disease control, the unidentified diphtheria carrier remained as a persistent threat among unimmunized communities.[35] In 1932, the discharge of hospital patients, deemed clinically cured through bacteriological examination, while still harbouring the diphtheria germs, prolonged at least two epidemics. Contemporary best practice recommended confirmation of two consecutive negative throat and naso-pharynx swabs before hospital discharge; however, this practice was not routine with all institutional medical officers, particularly those in charge of hospitals.[36]

Despite the success of active immunization, particularly in districts where diphtheria was formerly endemic, the position in Dublin, and in Limerick city, remained less than satisfactory. In Dublin, immunization schemes failed to stem the increasing incidence of diphtheria. During 1932, just over 2,000 children attended the municipal immunization centres, bringing the number treated over the previous four years to 3,789. Central health condemned the Dublin measures as being 'too limited in scope to combat the spread of disease in the capital' and again called on chief medical officer, Matt Russell, to organize a more widespread campaign of immunization in the city.[37] The complete lack of action by Limerick health authorities also received condemnation. In response, Limerick's chief medical officer, T. W. Moran, intimated that he planned to introduce systematic measures to combat diphtheria along the lines of the Cork model, which he expected to be adopted by Limerick Corporation 'sometime during 1933'.[38]

By 1933, efforts to combat diphtheria in the Free State had brought home two things to central health. The first was that the type of diphtheria experienced throughout the Free State was severe, and secondly, that immunization appeared to be the best weapon against it. The DLG&PH *Report* for 1933–34 states:

The extinction of communicable diseases may be regarded as the primary aim of preventive medicine and although the final triumph must still be regarded as remote, there is every reason to hope that in time a measure of control will be established which will result in

35 DLG&PH, *Report 1932–33*, 205–07.
36 Department of Local Government and Public Health, *Report 1933–34* (Stationery Office, Dublin), 224–25.
37 DLG&PH, *Report, 1932–33*, 45.
38 DLG&PH, *Report, 1932–33*, 203–05.

almost complete eradication of diseases such as Typhoid, Typhus, Scarlatina and Diphtheria.[39]

While the incidence of typhus and typhoid reduced to figures that gave central health 'reason to hope for their ultimate disappearance', the continued increase in the incidence of diphtheria was 'somewhat disturbing'. A departmental report for 1933 lamented, 'it is a matter of regret to record a marked increase in the number of cases of diphtheria notified to the department for the period under review'.[40] Some 3,369 cases occurred during 1933, including 1,681 cases recorded in the County Boroughs, comprised in the main by 1,073 cases from Dublin, and 445 from Limerick.

The 418 diphtheria fatalities recorded during 1933 was the highest number recorded since the inception of the Free State. Although a gradual decline in case fatalities occurred year on year to 1925, the subsequent eight years witnessed a steady increase. In fact, figures for 1933 represented an increase of 95 fatalities over the average annual diphtheria fatalities recorded for the previous five years. Almost 50 per cent of fatalities recorded during 1933 occurred in the county boroughs, with Dublin city alone accounting for 110, or 26 per cent of all diphtheria related fatalities for the year. This figure represented a shockingly high diphtheria mortality rate of 26 per 100,000 of the population, as compared with a national average of 14 per 100,000. In light of these figures, central health again urged Dublin health authorities to adopt a more effective system of immunization against diphtheria and to endeavour to bring home to the population of the city the necessity for having children immunized, particularly children aged 12 years and under. Although the Dublin public health department remonstrated that immunization clinics were in operation in the city since 1930, central health advised that figures relating to diphtheria morbidity and mortality in the city suggested that the municipal public health response 'had not been very satisfactory'.[41]

Similarly, an unsatisfactory public health intervention in Limerick city and county resulted in the highest incidence and case fatality rate recorded there for the previous six years. In Limerick city alone, 445 cases occurred during 1933, and municipal public health interventions there were, according to central health, 'outstandingly bad'. Despite the adoption of active immunization in Limerick during 1933, the diphtheria epidemic of the previous year continued unchecked. Central health concluded that in

39 DLG&PH, *Report 1933–34*, 38–39.
40 DLG&PH, *Report 1933–34*, 38–39.
41 DLG&PH, *Report 1933–34*, 51.

spite of the precautions undertaken, 'Limerick showed the need for entire re-organisation of its health services, none of which are satisfactory'.[42]

In the Northern District, Winslow Sterling-Berry reported that diphtheria of a severe type remained 'prevalent all over the district' and that notified cases required 'large and frequent doses of anti-diphtheritic serum to combat them'. On a brighter note, he observed that 'largely due to the excellent propaganda work of county medical officers', parents and teachers now demanded immunization services in areas where the disease was prevalent.[43] Sterling-Berry stressed that in districts where medical officers vigorously pursued immunization schemes, its value had been apparent. However, he lamented that some counties under his charge had yet to appoint a medical officer, which denied a large proportion of children under his supervision the advantages of 'our latest measure of prophylaxes'. Central health shared his concerns. Pointing to international evidence, the department asserted that in districts where children under five years of age were left without protection from diphtheria, it was possible to immunize 50 per cent of the school-going population without making 'any appreciable impression on the attack rate for diphtheria in the schools themselves'.[44]

The success associated with established immunization schemes, coupled with parental demand for access to immunization services, did much to lull the reticence of medical officers in districts still without an immunization scheme. In the winter of 1932, an acute outbreak in Caherciveen, County Kerry, prompted the inception of an immunization scheme there. Every child under 10 years of age, 1,347 in total, received full immunization treatment. In the following year, just three cases befell the area. In County Galway, immunization work was reportedly 'energetically carried on', and for the two years to 1933, almost 5,000 children presented for treatment. In addition, partial schemes sprang into operation in Carlow Dispensary District, County Carlow, Cavan and Ballinagh Dispensary Districts, County Cavan, Glin District, County Limerick, Tullamore Urban District, County Offaly, and in some districts of County Wexford.[45] In contrast, in areas such as Cashel Rural District, which endured recurrent epidemics, calls to inaugurate an immunization scheme went unheeded, as the local board of health had failed to appoint a full-time medical officer to the district.[46]

By 1934, intensive anti-diphtheria campaigns were operational in the

42 DLG&PH, *Report 1933–34*, 224–25.
43 DLG&PH, *Report 1933–34*, 51.
44 Edward. S. Godfrey, 'Study in the epidemiology of diphtheria in relation to active immunization of certain age groups', *American Journal of Public Health*, Vol. 22, No. 3 (March 1932), 237.
45 DLG&PH, *Report 1933–34*, 55.
46 DLG&PH, *Report 1933–34*, 224–25.

majority of districts possessing a full-time medical officer, and central health deemed the resultant decrease in incidence and mortality during the year as 'very gratifying'. The department acknowledged that, 'The decrease was in no small measure due to the reduction in the number of susceptible [children], which has resulted from the vigorous immunization campaign carried out by the county medical officers of health'.[47] The rollout of full-time medical officers, and the compulsory duty to notify disease outbreaks, has left a statistical record which for the first time comes close to an accurate representation of the prevalence of the principal epidemic diseases in the Free State. In the case of diphtheria, prevalence of the disease appears to increase dramatically from 1928–34, increasing from less than 1,000 cases during 1928 to almost 3,500 cases during 1934.[48] If we consider that 25 per cent of counties remained without a medical officer until 1936, then it may be reasonable to posit that the incidence of diphtheria in the Free State was closer to 4,600 cases annually. If we transpose this figure to the pre-vaccine era and factor in a case fatality rate of between 30–40 per cent, then the suggestion in chapter one that diphtheria fatalities in Ireland during the nineteenth century numbered between 1,500 and 2,500 annually begins to hold some credence.

For the seven years to 1934, the anti-diphtheria public health intervention conclusively demonstrated the value of active immunization as a preventive measure. Central health continued to promote the adoption of 'continuous and systematic [...] vigorous and intensive immunization schemes' with a view to establishing 'a population actively immune to diphtheria'.[49] The department directed every medical officer in the state to secure, and to have available at all times, a supply of diphtheria antitoxin from an official supplier, and urged them to keep their stock constantly renewed. While the department maintained a focus on prevention, they continued to promote passive immunity by inoculation and advised general practitioners and dispensary doctors to administer antitoxin to confirmed diphtheria cases at the earliest opportunity, and in large doses.[50]

Incidence of diphtheria diminished further during 1935. During the year, 3,091 cases occurred, down from 3,379 and 3,292 cases recorded during 1933 and 1934 respectively. The reducing national figures recorded over the three years to 1935 was influenced, in the main, by a substantial and sustained decrease in the county boroughs, where the most concentrated immuni-zation schemes were in operation. In Dublin city, a much-intensified scheme

47 Department of Local Government and Public Health, *Report 1934–35* (Stationery Office, Dublin), 224.
48 DLG&PH, *Reports, 1928–34*.
49 Department of Local Government and Public Health, *Report 1934–35* (Stationery Office), 65.
50 DLG&PH, *Report 1934–35*, 65.

influenced a reduction in morbidity from 1,073 cases in 1933, to 936 cases in 1935, and was accompanied by a decrease in case fatalities from 110 to 91 over the corresponding period.[51]

While notable reductions also occurred in Limerick and Waterford during 1935, the sustained decrease in Cork city was deemed by central health as being 'little short of dramatic'.[52] Here, incidence fell by more than 50 per cent, and case fatalities fell from 16 to just five, in a city where 100 annual diphtheria fatalities had previously been a more usual feature of the statistical record. In Cork city, Jack Saunders, was hopeful that 'granted full co-operation', his preventive scheme would reduce incidence and mortality even further. Central health had high praise for Saunders's work but remained largely unimpressed by his Dublin counterpart Matt Russell. For the five years to 1935, almost 47,000 children presented for immunization treatment in Dublin, though over the corresponding period, 54,200 new-borns were registered in the city, meaning that 'a large proportion of Dublin children remained unprotected against the dreaded scourge of diphtheria'.[53]

Anti-diphtheria Immunization in Dublin

In 1929, chief medical officer, Matt Russell, reported a substantial increase in diphtheria in Dublin. Russell insisted that his public health department operated 'a well-equipped disinfection station' and that the city had 'adequate hospital accommodation for the isolation of patients'. However, he conceded that these services failed to make any satisfactory impression on the incidence of diphtheria in the city.[54] Russell joined the Dublin public health department in 1911 as assistant to Sir Charles Cameron, who he succeeded in 1921 to become Dublin's first full-time municipal medical officer. Shortly after his appointment, Russell had travelled to America as a guest of the Rockefeller Foundation to study the advanced system of public health service provision in practice there and in particular, to study advances in preventive medicine.[55] Despite central health's backing, and legislation empowering

---

51 Although the results achieved in Dublin paled in comparison to those achieved in Cork, London public health authorities pointed to Dublin as an immunization model to emulate. See Max Sorsby, 'A note on diphtheria immunization in London', *British Medical Journal* (1 October 1938), 701–03.

52 Department of Local Government and Public Health, *Report 1935–36* (Stationery Office, Dublin), 55.

53 DLG&PH, *Report 1935–36*, 55.

54 *British Medical Journal* (13 September 1930), 444.

55 C. O'Brien, 'In memoriam, Matthew John Russell', *Irish Journal of Medical Science*, April 1956, 190.

sanitary authorities, and medical officers, to test children for susceptibility
to diphtheria infection and to administer protective agents where necessary,
it seems clear that as late as 1930, public health service provision in Dublin,
like their British counterparts, remained mired in sanitarian ideology.[56]

In May 1929, Dr Ray O'Meara, Rockefeller Foundation Fellow in Public
Health, contacted Russell with a view to investigating the prevalence of
diphtheria carriers among Dublin schoolchildren. As traditional methods of
disease prevention made little or no impact on the incidence of diphtheria in
the city, Russell pledged his full support and that of the school medical officer,
Dr Mary O'Leary. In the autumn of 1929, O'Meara began an examination
of 'unselected and apparently healthy children' attending schools in districts
throughout the city.[57]

O'Meara's investigation focused on three factors which determined the
prevalence of diphtheria in a community: the presence of the virulent
diphtheria bacillus, the susceptible individual, and the predisposing cause.
O'Meara's study emphasized the belief that knowledge of the diphtheria
carrier rate could provide a reliable index of the risk of exposure to
infection, and if high, might explain to some extent a high endemic survival
of diphtheria in a community.[58] He determined to classify carriers of the
diphtheria bacillus on anatomical grounds, as throat carriers, nose carriers,
ear carriers, and less frequently, other parts of the body such as the outer
genitals may carry the bacillus. For practical reasons the Dublin study was
limited to throat carriers and nose carriers only, as O'Meara considered these
cases to be 'by far of greatest significance when considering the propagation
of the disease'.

Over a period of twelve months, O'Meara made weekly visits to schools
throughout Dublin city where he examined 50 children on each visit.
He took both throat and nasal swabs from each child. Each week, 100
swabs were subjected to a rigorous bacteriological process ensuring: (1) the
culturing of the diphtheria bacilli; (2) their identification by microscopically
examination; (3) the confirmation of microscopically observations by fermentation reactions; and (4) the separation into non-virulent and virulent types
of diphtheria by animal inoculation.[59] O'Meara's study of 5,000 Dublin
schoolchildren suggested that 50 children, or 5 per cent of those tested, gave
positive cultures of morphological diphtheria bacilli, 46 per cent of which
were of the virulent type. When applied to the city's entire school population,

56 The Public Health (Infectious Disease) Regulations, 1929, Amendment No. 4.
57 R. A. Q. O'Meara, 'The prevalence of diphtheria carriers among Dublin school
    children', *Irish Journal of Medical Science*, Vol. 6, No. 3 (March 1931), 125–33.
58 O'Meara, *IJMS*, 1931, 127.
59 O'Meara, *IJMS*, 1931, 127.

the results suggested that over 3,000 Dublin schoolchildren were diphtheria carriers, 1,400 of whom were carriers of virulent diphtheria bacilli.

Analysis of O'Meara's findings shows that the carrier rate among boys was 4.5 per cent, with an associated virulent carrier rate of 1.6 per cent; however, among girls the rate was substantially higher, registering 5.6 per cent and 3.1 per cent respectively.[60] Research undertaken by Von Sholly and Wilcox involving 1,000 children from tenement districts in New York revealed a carrier rate of 5.6 per cent and a virulent rate of 1.8 per cent.[61] An investigation undertaken by Guthrie, Gelien, and Moss relating to 1,217 schoolchildren in Baltimore, Maryland, established a diphtheria carrier rate of 3.61 per cent and a virulent rate of 0.67 per cent.[62] In Berlin, Pieper examined 36,824 children, of whom just 1.0 per cent gave positive cultures, and in London, Graham Forbes examination of 12,017 children revealed a carrier rate of 5.9 per cent and a virulent rate averaging 2.95 per cent.[63] Taken as a whole, the carrier rates identified among Dublin schoolchildren were at the high end of the scale, but mirrored rates found in many other districts. However, a comparison of virulent rates of diphtheria in these districts suggests that Dublin registered an average rate of 2.3 per cent, one of the highest virulent rates recorded and second only to London at 2.95 per cent. O'Meara concluded, 'It would seem from the results that the carrier is not to be regarded as a rarity, but as commonplace. It is the case of diphtheria rather than the carrier, which is the rarity'.[64]

In her investigation into the health of Dublin schoolchildren, school medical officer, Dr Mary O'Leary, observed that the most frequently found defect was the most difficult to remedy – overcrowding.[65] In older and invariably densely populated districts of the city, schoolhouses were largely unsuitable buildings such as old churches, and in some instances, church basements. Although new schools built to accommodate 2,000 children were springing up on the outskirts of the city, over 4,000 children sought admission.

In general, schools were without playground space or covered portions for wet days. Classrooms were dark, lightless, and airless spaces where children

60 O'Meara, *IJMS*, 1931, 130.
61 Anna Von Sholly and Harriet Wilcox, 'A contribution to the statistics of the presence of diphtheria bacilli in apparently normal throats', *Journal of Infectious Diseases*, Vol. 4 (1907), 337.
62 C. Guthrie, J. Gilien, and W. L. Moss, 'Diphtheria Bacillus Carriers', 2nd Communication, *Bulletin; John Hopkins Hospital*, Vol. 31 (1920), 388.
63 J. Graham Forbes, 'The problem of the diphtheria carrier in London children of school age', *Public Health*, XXXVI (1923), 323.
64 O'Meara, *Irish Journal of Medical Science* (1931), 132.
65 Mary M. O'Leary, 'A survey of the health of the Dublin school child', *Irish Journal of Medical Science* (April 1931), 155–61.

sat for hours 'packed together like dolls on the shelves of a crowded toy shop'.[66] Inadequate government funding, and inadequate voluntary contributions, ensured that many schools remained bereft of heating arrangements, and in most cases cleaned just once a year. No provision existed for washing, and outside taps supplied drinking water to a single metal cup shared by hundreds of children. A consideration of O'Leary's report in light of O'Meara's findings brought the seriousness of the situation home to Russell and the Dublin public health authorities, and with it, a realization that reliance on traditional sanitarian methods of disease control would require a radical reappraisal.

In July 1930, a conference organized by the DLG&PH and convened by Minister Richard Mulcahy, invited delegates from every health board in the Free State to an assembly at the Mansion House, Dublin. The conference gave newly appointed medical officers a national platform from which to promote innovative public health interventions. Jack Saunders, Cork city, and John Musgrave, County Louth, addressed attendees on the economic benefits of adopting preventive measures in health and administration. Both men asserted that preventive medicine undoubtedly 'raised the general standard of health and the happiness of the people', but also that when the question of the cost of preventive measures was measured against the cost of hospitalization, 'the former proved to be cheaper'.[67]

During 1930, increased rates of diphtheria again confronted Russell. It is unclear whether Saunders and Musgrave had convinced Russell of the benefits of active immunization, or whether he was compelled to act by central health, but shortly after the Mansion House meeting, Russell began to vocalize the view that the only effective means of controlling diphtheria lay with immunization. With the approval of the local government board, Russell appointed Dr Denis Hanley of Cork Street Fever Hospital to oversee arrangements for the rollout of a limited anti-diphtheria immunization scheme in the city. This took the form of a weekly two-hour session at the Carnegie Centre, Lord Edward Street (now Dame Street). Dublin Corporation provided £400 in their estimates to cover the cost of the service; however, this allocation was also to cover the cost of supplying diphtheria antitoxin to 'suitable children's hospitals where the work of immunization might be undertaken'.[68] Welcoming the launch of the Dublin campaign, city commissioner, Dr Dwyer, optimistically stated:

For some time past, the growing numbers of diphtheria cases have been causing considerable alarm to the Medical Officer of Health and

66 O'Leary, *Irish Journal of Medical Science* (1931), 155.
67 'Keystone of public health', *Irish Times*, 9 July 1930.
68 'The prevention of diphtheria', *Irish Times*, 3 September 1930.

the Commissioners. This clinic has been started, and we have hopes that, not only will the great volume of human suffering be avoided, but also the ever-increasing cost of the treatment of fever cases, which fall directly on the rates, will be curtailed.[69]

Analysis of statistics at Denis Hanley's disposal brought him to the conclusion that while the greatest incidence of diphtheria occurred among school-going children, mortality fell heaviest on the pre-school age group. In a bid to protect this most vulnerable section of the population, Hanley focused the Dublin campaign exclusively on children of pre-school age. His aim was to achieve at least 75 per cent coverage among pre-school children thereby 'automatically supplying schools with already protected children'.[70] This approach sought to negate the necessity of conducting immunization schemes in the city schools. However, this tight-fisted approach to disease control was doomed before it began. In the period May 1930 to October 1934, 14,802 pre-school children presented for treatment. Although 12,980 children completed the full course of treatment, this represented little over 10 per cent of the city's susceptible child population. Despite the extension of immunization services to two sessions per week at the Carnegie Centre, and weekly clinics at Lourdes House, Buckingham Street, and St Andrews, Mount Street, Hanley regarded the public response to the initiative as 'very disappointing'.[71]

The Dublin scheme was both frugal and restricted in scope, and did little to stem the rise of diphtheria cases in the city. For the years 1931–33, notifications more than doubled to 1,095, representing an increase of 100 per cent over the decennial average for the previous decade.[72] As the majority of infected children presented at the city hospitals, Russell lamented that recorded notifications reflected an accurate account of the prevalence of diphtheria in the city. Although Russell took some solace in the 'accuracy of the reporting', he was slow to acknowledge the complete failure of his intervention. Instead, he pointed the finger at parents and accused them of 'failing in their responsibility to their children if they did not take fuller advantage of the immunization clinics established in the city'.[73]

69 'Dublin city commissioners: The governments successful experiment', *Irish Times*, 23 August 1930.
70 D. F. Hanley, 'Anti-diphtheria immunization', *Irish Journal of Medical Science*, Vol. 12, No. 9 (September 1937), 578–85.
71 Matthew J. Russell, *Report on the state of public health in the City of Dublin for the year 1931* (Dublin, 1932), 28.
72 Matthew J. Russell, *Report on the state of public health in the City of Dublin for the year 1933* (Dublin, 1934), 22.
73 Russell, *Dublin Report 1933*, 23.

Figures relating to diphtheria for 1933 show that 30 per cent of cases were aged four years or younger, 17 per cent aged 15 or older, and 53 per cent occurred within the 5–14 age bracket. This suggests that municipal immunization services had not been available to 70 per cent of children who contracted diphtheria during 1933, which renders Russell's charge against parents untenable. Furthermore, 50 per cent of cases occurred outside school-going age groups. This suggests that although the school environment played a significant role in propagating diphtheria, it was not the only predisposing factor in Dublin. Monthly records charting diphtheria cases during 1933 show that the disease did peak during October and November. However, incidence during the summer months show no sign of diminution and it seems clear that diphtheria was prevalent in the city throughout the year.

Analysis of diphtheria mortality during 1933 reveals that the vast majority of fatalities, in fact, all but one, occurred in children aged under 14 years: half were four years or younger. Among this pre-school age group, fatalities distributed evenly between girls and boys, each registering 27 fatalities. However, analysis of fatalities in the 5–14 age groups shows that diphtheria fell heaviest on girls, who accounted for 62 per cent of cases, and 74 per cent of case fatalities in this age bracket.[74]

Russell conceded that the presence of diphtheria 'carriers' in overcrowded schools was 'a positive menace to other children and playmates who are not immune to this infection'. However, as fatalities were more prevalent among pre-school children, the public health intervention maintained a focus there.[75] The idea behind this approach sought not only to address high diphtheria mortality among the pre-school group, but also to provide immunological protection to children who were about to become exposed to the known risks of school life, particularly in respect to diphtheria. Although 10,273 children attended municipal immunization clinics during 1933, fewer than 3,467 completed the full course of treatment. As immunization services were available to pre-school children only, it is possible to deduce that the numbers treated represented 7.6 per cent of the city's pre-school population and little more than 2.8 per cent of the city's general child population. These figures fell far short of the 75 per cent target protection rate Russell aspired to.

Despite the shortcomings of the Dublin campaign, and the somewhat indifferent public response, a 9 per cent reduction in incidence ensued during 1934. In those 15 years and older, 182 cases occurred, representing 18 per cent of cases and a slight increase on the previous year. Among the

74 Russell, *Dublin Report 1933*, 27.
75 Russell, *Dublin Report 1933*, 28.

5–14 age group, 500 cases occurred representing 51 per cent of cases and a slight decrease on the previous year. Among those aged four years and younger, 301 cases occurred, representing 31 per cent of cases, and a slight increase on the previous year.[76]

While the percentage incidence in the three age groups deviated little from previous years, analysis of diphtheria mortality recorded during 1934 reveals a notable alteration. While case mortality rates among those aged 15 and older remained unchanged at around 1 per cent, case mortality rates among school-going children aged 5–14 years increased substantially from 49 per cent in 1933, to 55 per cent in 1934. Conversely, case mortality among the pre-school population, those aged four years and younger, saw a dramatic reduction from 50 per cent in 1933, to 39 per cent during 1934. Considering that the Dublin anti-diphtheria immunization programme had concentrated exclusively on this age group, it must be reasonable to assert that the dramatic diminution in case fatalities among pre-school children was linked directly to the focus maintained on this section of the population.[77]

It had taken four years to achieve this minor victory in the war on diphtheria, and an enthused Russell pleaded for 'the whole-hearted co-operation of the citizen [...] as without it epidemic diphtheria would maintain its deadly course'. Dublin health authorities advised parents that children 'can and should be immunised' and that 'maximum benefit' and 'minimum discomfort' followed treatment in the first year of life. Intensified propaganda efforts met with some success, in that the number of pre-school children who completed treatment during 1934 almost doubled to 5,614. This brought the total number of children who completed treatment over the four years to 1934 to 10,984. This number still represented fewer than 10 per cent of all pre-school children in the city, and the fact that over 90 per cent remained vulnerable to the ravages of diphtheria remained a cause of frustration among the city's public health officials. Notwithstanding, Russell stuck to his initial plan, consoling his colleagues in the public health department with the thought that even if the slow rate of progress in pre-school immunizations was maintained for some years, that protection would eventually be secured for more than 60 per cent of pre-school children.[78] He stated: 'Then, with the school population being recruited from this relatively highly-protected group, our entire child population will benefit by the disappearance of epidemic diphtheria'.[79]

---

76 Matthew J. Russell, *Report on the state of public health in the City of Dublin for the year 1934* (Dublin, 1935), 24.
77 Russell, *Dublin Report 1934*, 24.
78 Russell, *Dublin Report 1934*, 32–33.
79 Russell, *Dublin Report 1934*, 33.

This reasoning made little sense, and more disturbingly, Russell seemed quite willing to allow over 76,000 schoolchildren to remain exposed to the dangers associated with diphtheria. In a city with a child population of 121,850, and a live birth rate of 11,500 infants per year, the public health response to diphtheria in Dublin was going to need another radical rethink. The aspirational, but elusive, 75 per cent protection rate among pre-school children in theory obviated the necessity to undertake immunization programmes in the city schools, as Russell hoped that this approach, at some time in the future, would automatically supply city schools with immunized children. However, the gradual acceptance that diphtheria was in fact endemic in Dublin brought with it a realization that anti-diphtheria immunization schemes in the city schools would not only be necessary, but essential.

J. C. Saunders Anti-diphtheria Intervention in Cork City

An outbreak of diphtheria in Cork city in 1930 was, and remains, one of the worst outbreaks in the country, and possibly Europe. The heaviest incidence fell on children aged 10 years and younger. Analysis of reported cases shows seven infants, 159 children aged 1–5 years, 207 children aged 5–10 years, 88 children aged 10–15 years, 49 cases aged 15–20, and 114 cases in those aged 20 and older. Characteristically, schoolchildren suffered most severely.[80]

During the 1930 epidemic, hospitals recorded that 18 per cent of cases occurred in people aged 20 years and older. Occurrence among this age group was 'an unusual feature of the disease' and chief medical officer, Jack Saunders, considered the figure 'abnormally high'. On further investigation Saunders discovered that two cases notified, in people aged over sixty years, were not in fact diphtheria and it seemed likely that many notified cases had been misdiagnosed. New-born infants are generally Schick negative due to immunity contracted while in the womb, but the level of immunity steadily diminishes over twelve months.[81] The fact that hospitals notified seven cases of infant diphtheria bolstered Saunders's suspicions of misdiagnosis, as occurrence in this age group was also an unusual feature of the disease.[82]

It was not possible for the public health department to check admissions and diagnosis of hospitalized cases; however, it was possible for them

80 J. C. Saunders, *Report of the Medical Officer of Health for the year 1930* (Eagle Printing, Cork, 1931).
81 Sir Frank McFarlane Burnet and David O. White, *Natural history of infectious disease* (Cambridge, 1972), 198.
82 Saunders, *Report 1930*, 16.

to monitor cases attending the municipal public health clinic, and those notified to the department as suffering from diphtheria. Examination of 50 such children failed to confirm diagnoses in 19 cases.[83] When applied to total notifications for 1930, it appears that misdiagnosis had occurred in over one third of notified cases. Analysis of the 63 case fatalities reveals that 57.82 per cent were under four years old, 34.37 per cent were between 5–10 years, 6.25 per cent were aged 10–15 years, and 1.56 per cent were aged over twenty years. The startling fact was that 92.29 per cent of diphtheria fatalities occurred in children under ten years old.[84]

Traditional methods utilized to stem the spread of diphtheria in Ireland and Britain consisted of notification, prompt isolation of the patient, a period of quarantine for contacts with exclusion from school of all children, steam disinfection of bedding, apparel and other clothing used by the patient, and 'disinfection by fumigating the patients apartment'.[85] However, because diphtheria is a specific microorganism, traditional methods of preventing its propagation achieved only limited success.

The principal factor in the propagation of diphtheria is the 'carrier', a person who may not display any symptoms of the disease themselves but who may act as a source of infection, posing a threat to the community as a whole. Those who recover from diphtheric infection continue to harbour germs of the disease in their throat and remain infective for a period after convalescence. On returning to school, the apparently healthy child may continue to act as a reservoir of infection, and close contact with classmates ensured continued propagation of the disease. In a bid to combat this, convalescing children underwent a nose and throat swab and were required to return two successive negative swabs before discharge from hospital.

At certain times of the year, owing to a lack of hospital accommodation, it was not possible to hospitalize infectious patients for the recommended amount of time, and city manager Philip Monaghan conceded that 'this difficulty arose particularly in the case of diphtheria patients'.[86] Neither of the city hospitals tasked with treating infectious disease was under Saunders's control and of 600 beds available in one hospital, only two accommodated children. The second institution was, according to Henry Parish, of the Wellcome Laboratories, under the charge of 'an old doctor who was a failure in general practice', who refused to take blood for examination 'and does

83 Saunders, *Report 1930*, 14.
84 Saunders, *Report 1930*, 15.
85 J. C. Saunders, *Report of the Medical Officer of Health for the year 1931* (Eagle Printing, Cork, 1932), 23.
86 'Diphtheria patients in Cork: Insufficient hospital accommodation', *Irish Times*, 9 May 1929.

not seem to know how to do it'.[87] Parish also noted that facilities to perform virulence tests of serums and prophylactics were not available in Cork. The bacteriologist at University College Cork had on occasion performed a subcutaneous test, and Saunders relied on the Wellcome laboratories in Beckenham, London, to undertake his tests, and to determine bacteriological diagnosis in contested diphtheria cases.[88] Saunders acknowledged that the city hospitals were working to full capacity, that longer detention of infectious patients was not practicable and that 'one could not look to them further to check the spread of disease'.[89]

Saunders recognized the steadily rising number of diphtheria cases during April and May 1929 as an ominous sign that the onset of an epidemic was imminent. He was equally convinced that the city was not equipped with adequate resources to deal with such a visitation.[90] He summed up the situation thus:

> The position of affairs was apparently very gloomy. We had the highest incidence of diphtheria in the British Isles. A large number of children died from the disease every year. Our hospitals were taxed to their fullest capacity and the overcrowded nature of many of our schools favoured the propagation of the disease. Large sums of public money were being expended annually in treating the disease and if reliance was to be continued in existent methods still more expenditure would have to be incurred to check its spread. There was, fortunately at our disposal a simpler and more-speedy method of preventing the occurrence of diphtheria.[91]

Saunders was concerned that an epidemic period was an unsuitable time for the introduction of an immunization scheme. The development of post-treatment immunity required a period of six months to pass, and it was certain that some treated children would succumb to the disease before developing full protection. There was a danger that such cases would create a negative impression of anti-diphtheria immunization. Saunders concluded that there were only two options at his disposal, 'to adopt a laissez faire attitude and allow the disease to run its course or, to implement a scheme of immunization'.[92] The history of diphtheria in Cork city, particularly since 1919, demonstrated that all available methods failed to check the disease.

87 WF/M/GB/01/37/01. Henry Parish, Confidential Notes on visit to Cork.
88 Henry Parish, Confidential Notes on visit to Cork.
89 Saunders, *Report 1931*, 25.
90 Saunders, *Report 1931*, 26.
91 Saunders, *Report 1931*, 25.
92 Saunders, *Report 1931*, 26.

There was no prospect that the disease would end if 'let to run its course'. City hospitals were 'old and inadequate' and cases of cross infection were so prevalent that diphtheria attained the moniker 'hospital throat'.[93] Children were dying from diphtheria, and there was 'a marked uneasiness all over the city in regard to it'. Saunders concluded:

> The previous history of the disease gave no indication that there was any finality within sight for years to come [...] based on the experiences of other cities, the only hope of amelioration lay in the widespread application of immunization and for this reason it was decided to incur the risks [...] in the interest of the community as distinct from that of the individual [...] it only remained to place at the disposal of the citizens the means of protecting their children against this very dangerous disease, the hazards of which were so much greater in this city than practically any other in Europe.[94]

In May 1929, Saunders asked Cork city council for £300 to be included in the estimates for the year to fund a special diphtheria immunization scheme in the city, to 'facilitate parents who wished to have their children rendered immune to the disease'.[95] Saunders argued that the cost of treating each case of diphtheria amounted to £6, and cost the city £2,000 annually. He predicted that if the disease continued unchecked, this amount would double during 1930, and even more expenditure would be required to address the lack of hospital accommodation for diphtheria patients.[96] Saunders suggested that at a cost of 2s. 6d. to 3s. per child, the prevention of diphtheria through immunization would prove far more economical than the projected cost of treating the disease.[97] The council agreed, and Saunders made arrangements for the opening of an anti-diphtheria immunization campaign.[98]

In the absence of legislation compelling parents to submit children for immunization treatment, Saunders launched a public campaign promoting active immunization. In June 1929, he received an invitation to address the local Rotary Club on the subject, and the event received coverage in the local and national press. This was followed by an address to school teachers in the city and county, active canvassing of sanitary inspectors, school nurses, and health visitors, the exhibition of lantern slides and 'cinematographic pictures'

93 Farmar, *Patients, potions, physicians*, 139.
94 Saunders, *Report 1931*, 25–26.
95 'Cork plan to combat disease', *Irish Times*, 29 April 1929.
96 'Scheme to fight disease', *Irish Times*, 10 June 1929.
97 *Irish Times*, 29 April 1929.
98 *Irish Times*, 10 June 1929.

in local cinemas, and the distribution of 5,000 pamphlets, *Information to parents re Diphtheria Immunization*.[99]

On 6 June 1929, the Cork anti-diphtheria immunization scheme began in earnest. At the public health clinic on Parnell Place, Saunders, assisted by Dr O'Sullivan and Nurse Lyndon of the School Medical Service, administered anti-diphtheria immunization treatment to 100 children, selected by the Child Welfare League.[100] It is not clear whether these children were selected from private or institutional settings and the issue of parental consent, or indeed informed consent is absent from the surviving historical record. However, according to Henry Parish, the first name, which appeared in the Cork city immunization register, is that of Saunders's own daughter, who he insisted on being the first child to receive immunization treatment 'in order to gain the confidence of mothers'. In the early weeks of the campaign, queues of mothers and their children extended down two flights of stairs and into the street at Parnell Place, and crowds were reportedly so large at times that they were 'regulated by policemen, like a cinema queue'.[101]

The high attendances at the public health clinic were encouraging; however, expansion of the scheme would require not only the support of parents, but also teachers. At a meeting of the Cork branch of the Irish National Teachers Organisation (INTO), Saunders discussed the process of treating diphtheria with the city's national-school teachers. Concerns were raised as to the safety and effectiveness of the immunization process and the possible danger of post-immunization disease supervening.[102] Understandably, those concerned drew parallels between anti-diphtheria immunization and the already established compulsory smallpox vaccination scheme, which some held responsible for cases of post-vaccination encephalitis, and a number of fatalities.[103] Saunders conceded that the cause of post-vaccination 'sleepy sickness' was under investigation, but he stressed that anti-diphtheria immunization was 'an entirely different process' used on 1,000,000 children in New York alone, 'without a single ill effect'. Despite some reservations, the INTO members supported expenditure on the prevention of 'this terrible disease' as 'money well spent' and promised Saunders their 'hearty co-operation' in support of the scheme.[104]

By the end of 1929, 1,802 children presented for immunization treatment with Burroughs Wellcome toxin-antitoxin mixture (TAM). In order to

99   CC&CA, CP/C/CM/PH/A/30, June–October 1929.
100 'A woman's social diary; Cork anti-diphtheria scheme', *Cork Examiner*, 14 June 1929.
101 Parish, Notes on visit to Cork.
102 'Diphtheria: Lecture to Cork teachers', *Cork Examiner*, 17 June 1929.
103 Charles Armstrong, 'Post-vaccination encephalitis', *Annals of Internal Medicine*, Vol. 5, No. 3 (1 September 1931), 333–37.
104 *Cork Examiner*, 17 June 1929.

monitor proceedings, Saunders undertook almost all of the immunization work himself and reportedly treated up to '400 children at one session single-handed'.[105] A survey undertaken in April 1930, found that of those treated, 12 children subsequently contracted diphtheria. When Saunders investigated these cases, he found that four of the infected children had not completed a full course of treatment (three received one injection, and one received two injections). In three cases, a period of less than four months had elapsed since receiving treatment, and in three further cases, he could not confirm diagnosis.[106] Saunders confirmed diagnosis in the two remaining children, which equated to an incidence rate of 0.11 per cent among treated children.

During the same period, 298 cases of diphtheria were notified amongst the general child population of the city (recorded as being 22,605) an equivalent incidence rate of 1.31 per cent. These early results indicated that immunized children were substantially less at risk of contracting diphtheria than those who remained untreated. In addition, utilization of the Schick test at the public health clinic showed that the proportion of children found to be Schick positive and therefore susceptible to diphtheria before immunization treatment was 78.29 per cent. Post-treatment Schick tests performed on children who completed the full course of treatment showed that only 6.58 per cent returned a positive reaction. When these children received an extra dose of TAM and retested, the proportion of treated children subsequently testing positive fell to 0.25 per cent.[107]

Due to a special drive in the city schools, by the end of 1930 over 5,100 children received treatment, with 4,659, or one fifth of the total child population of the city having completed the full course. Saunders hoped that many thousands more children would have presented for treatment, but concurrent epidemics of measles and mumps forced a temporary suspension of immunization in the city schools.[108] An added complication was that the large number of diphtheria cases diagnosed during the year placed increased pressure on city hospitals, which resulted in continued premature discharge of patients.[109] Of 4,659 children who completed the full course of treatment, 11 subsequently developed diphtheria, representing an incidence rate of 0.23 per cent.

These post-treatment cases developed mild diphtheria symptoms; the severity of the disease modified by immunizing treatment. Of the 17,496 children who did not present for treatment, 461 cases of diphtheria occurred,

105 Parish, Notes on Cork visit.
106 Saunders, *Report 1930*, 18.
107 Saunders, *Report 1930*, 20.
108 'The health of Cork: City's high death rate', *Irish Times*, 4 June 1930.
109 'Corks share of sweepstake funds', *Irish Times*, 15 April 1931.

giving an equivalent incidence rate of 2.63 per cent. The results showed that the prevalence of diphtheria among unimmunized, and therefore susceptible children, was almost 12 times greater than among immunized children. Case mortality rates among immunized and non-immunized children were even more striking. In 1930, fatalities among untreated children numbered 64, while case fatalities among immunized children were nil.[110]

Initial results were positive. However, the use of TAM as an anti-diphtheria antigen had its drawbacks. Firstly, securing a desired 80–85 per cent negative Schick test result with TAM required a period of eight months to elapse after treatment. Secondly, a full course of immunization treatment with TAM necessitated up to five interactions between child and doctor: each child subjected to pre-treatment and post-treatment Schick tests, along with, at least three, and possibly four intramuscular injections.

Saunders's anti-diphtheria campaign garnered good public support, but the occurrence of 50 post-treatment cases threatened to undermine it. On admission to hospital, bacteriological examination failed to confirm diphtheria in 19 of these cases. Where post-treatment diphtheria did occur, the majority had not completed a full course of treatment.[111] The periodic occurrence of post-treatment cases, suspected or confirmed, undermined public confidence and acted as a major disincentive to parents to present their children for treatment. As a result, over 13 per cent of parents failed to return their children to complete a full course of anti-diphtheria immunization treatment.

This substantial 'desertion rate' did little to offset the severity of the epidemic. Over the previous eighteen months, 957 diphtheria cases occurred in the city. Ninety-eight children perished, and a growing number of partially treated children continued to contract diphtheria. From the trenches, Saunders began to consider the use of an alternative antigen, one that would induce immunization quicker and to a higher degree than TAM, administered in one injection, and free from unpleasant reactions.

110 Saunders, *Report 1930*, 20.
111 Saunders, *Report 1930*, 19.

4

Developing Burroughs Wellcome
Alum-Toxoid

A nti-diphtheria immunization combining Schick testing and active
immunization with Toxin-Antitoxin Mixture commenced in Britain
in 1920. However, the practice was restricted to residential institutions
in London, Birmingham, Bristol, Manchester, Edinburgh, Glasgow, and
Aberdeen, and supervised by local medical authorities, the Ministry of
Health, and personnel attached to the Wellcome Research Laboratories.[1]
From 1922 to 1925, active immunization with antitoxin extended to include
elementary schools in Edinburgh, Aberdeen, Birmingham, and Cardiff, and
to infant welfare centres in the London boroughs of Holborn, Westminster,
and Camberwell. However, antitoxin mixtures never found a commercial
outlet in Britain as health authorities there considered the serums 'potentially
unsafe'.[2] Reticence to adopt antitoxin on a mass scale in Britain lay with
the fact that the safety, or otherwise, of antitoxin, relied heavily on the
production of a neutralized toxin. Failure to adhere to this formula at the
production stage, or indeed any subsequent mishandling of toxin–antitoxin,
could and had proved to have lethal consequences.

In 1919, an error during the production of toxin–antitoxin in a Dallas
laboratory resulted in the production of a toxic mixture. Whether due to
inexperience or accident, the addition of toxin to the toxoid in two stages,
rather than the recommended one stage process, resulted in a Danyze
phenomenon, and the production of an unequal, un-neutralized mixture.
When the toxic mixture was utilized in an immunization scheme, 45 children
experienced severe reactions, and five fatalities ensued.[3] In 1924, in the
towns of Concord and Bridgewater, Massachusetts, a single bottle of toxin-

---

1 J. Graham Forbes, *The prevention of diphtheria* (London, 1927), 9.
2 Parish, *Immunization*, 147.
3 W. H. Park, 'Some important facts concerning active immunization against diphtheria',
   American Journal of Diseases of Children, Vol. 32, No. 5 (1926), 709–17.

antitoxin caused severe reactions in 40 children. Although many hundreds of children received treatment with serum from the same batch, health authorities discovered that the affected children all received serum from the same bottle.[4] Subsequently, William Park, found that the suspect bottle was stored below freezing point: thereby altering its chemical composition. Alternate freezing and thawing gave rise to a local concentration of the preservative Phenol, causing a destruction of the antitoxin, resulting in an unbalanced toxic mixture.[5]

In Europe, the administration of a local preparation, issued as toxin-antitoxin, resulted in six infant fatalities at a children's home in Baden, near Vienna, in 1925. In this case, an investigation conducted by the Hygienic Institute found that due to a laboratory error, technicians omitted to add the necessary antitoxin control, and the serum issued contained pure toxin only. In response to the Baden incident, the Austrian Ministry of Health suspended active immunization.[6] Although these incidents were largely avoidable, they were wholly unpalatable, and attracted severe criticisms of active immunization procedures. Notwithstanding, advocates of active immunization remained steadfast in their support, and the confidence of the American health authorities in particular remained largely unshaken. In Britain, Richard O'Brien, Director of the Wellcome Physiological Research Laboratory, urged the Ministry of Health against the commercialization of European and American produced toxin-antitoxin in Britain on the basis that these products were potentially unsafe.[7] Whether O'Brien's motives were genuinely altruistic or otherwise, the timing coincided with the efforts of his employers Burroughs Wellcome to develop their own brand of anti-diphtheria prophylactic for the British market.

At Wellcome Laboratories, Alexander Glenny produced a modified 'detoxicated' serum, or toxoid: a serum rendered harmless by the removal of toxin, without affecting efficacy. Glenny's discovery demonstrated that formalin used to clean bulk containers, when added to antitoxin, greatly reduced the minimum lethal dose value of the serum, while maintaining antigenicity.[8] Prior to the 1920s, Glenny confined the use of his de-toxicated serum to animals; however, in 1921 Wellcome put this new toxoid through a series of clinical tests with a view to its substitution in place of toxin-antitoxin. In November and December 1921, Dr Thomas Archibald undertook the first of these trials at Belvidere Fever Hospital,

4 Forbes, *Prevention of diphtheria*, 11.
5 Park, *American Journal of Diseases of Children*, 709–17.
6 Forbes, *Prevention of diphtheria*, 11–12.
7 H. J. Parish, *Victory with vaccines* (London, 1968), 91–93.
8 Parish, *Immunization*, 141.

Glasgow. Wellcome provided the serum free of charge and Archibald administered it to 181 staff and patients at Belvidere. The positive results achieved in Glasgow encouraged Wellcome, with Ministry of Health backing, to conduct further trials to obtain 'valuable independent evidence regarding the degree and duration of protection bestowed by British-made anti-diphtheria prophylactics'.[9] Between 1923 and 1927, O'Brien and his colleagues at Wellcome instituted and oversaw clinical trials of Glenny's toxoid-antitoxin mixture in a range of British residential institutions, where over 4,500 people were Schick tested, and over 1,400 received treatment with the experimental toxoid.[10]

The institutions involved in the trials included the Holborn Poor Law Schools, Mitcham; the Lambeth Poor Law Schools, West Norwood; Dr Barnardo's Home for Girls at Barkingside, Ilford; the naval training ship 'Exmouth' stationed off Grays, Essex; the naval training ship 'Cornwall' stationed off Gravesend, Kent; the Foundling Hospital while at Redhill, and Berkhamsted; the Rachel MacMillan School at Deptford and the Training School for Nurses at St Bartholomew's Hospital London.[11] Clinical research conducted in these institutions was, according to Henry Parish, 'the outcome of pressing invitations to control diphtheria outbreaks', and were overseen by medical officers on behalf of the Ministry of Health, who it was stated 'had no facilities to undertake immunization work themselves'.[12]

At Wellcome, Richard O'Brien regarded the results of the trials as 'thoroughly satisfactory' in preventing and controlling outbreaks of diphtheria, and resolved to take 'every opportunity provided for testing new techniques or variations of old ones'. In accordance with the indications provided by Glenny's research, who examined blood specimens to determine both the degree and duration of immunity of serums of differing chemical composition, Wellcome introduced two commercially available anti-diphtheria prophylactics in the form of toxoid-antitoxin mixture (TAM) in 1923 and TAF in 1927.[13] Ministry of Health officials, Sydney M. Copeman and W. A. Lothem, who facilitated and observed the trials, were reportedly 'fully satisfied' with the results, advised the Ministry to advocate this line of prevention, and urged its adoption by local authorities.[14]

9 R. A. O'Brien, 'Schick test and subsequent active immunization', *Proceedings of the Royal Society of Medicine*, Vol. 15 (1922); (Section on Epidemiology and State Medicine), 45–48.
10 O'Brien, *Royal Society of Medicine*, 1922, 48.
11 WF/M/H/08/10. Henry Parish, *The Wellcome Research Laboratories and immunization: A historical survey and personal memoir*, Chapters 7 to 9, c. 1970, Chapter 8; 2–3.
12 Parish, *A historical survey and personal memoir*, Chapter 8, 2–3.
13 Parish, *A historical survey and personal memoir*, Chapter 8, 5.
14 Forbes, *Prevention of diphtheria*, 31.

While a sanitarian ideology prevailed among British public health administrators, there is evidence also that a strong anti-vivisection and anti-vaccination lobby militated against the mass adoption of anti-diphtheria immunization in Britain. For instance, Richard O'Brien's intervention in Barnardo's Home for Girls was so successful in halting a diphtheria outbreak that 'a prominent representative of the staff' expressed their gratitude in a letter to *The Times*. The letter provoked an unexpected reaction from some of the home's patrons, who demanded 'a halt to experimentation on defenceless children', under penalty of discontinuing their subscriptions. Henry Parish later remarked; 'Wisely, there were no further letters to the press – and no more interruptions of the programme'.[15]

In 1928, the Ministry of Health made a commitment to test and immunize all English schoolchildren by the Schick method, and faced with increased prevalence of diphtheria that year, encouraged British education authorities to 'follow the lead of New York' in adopting immunization schemes. However, reports of immunization fatalities due to laboratory error deterred British authorities from arranging facilities to carry out immunization work. The Ministry of Health was forced to acknowledge that such recurring mishaps, only served to strengthen the already 'widespread objection to the adoption of any therapeutic measures involving the use of inoculation methods' in Britain.[16] As one contemporary observed, 'Progress marches slowly in England, for medical investigators have a full – the eager research worker may be inclined to say "overfull" sense of responsibility, and try the new thing with the greatest caution'.[17]

Immunization accidents in Texas and Massachusetts, both due to the negligence of laboratory technicians, had influenced the British government to introduce the Therapeutic Substances Act, 1925. This measure provided for the regulation of the manufacture, sale, and production of vaccines, sera, and other prophylactics, and introduced new requirements for biological testing of substances, where 'the potency of which cannot be adequately tested by chemical means'.[18] Subsequent fatal immunization accidents in Russia,[19] China,[20]

15 Parish, *A historical survey and personal memoir*, Chapter 8, 5.
16 Sydney Monckton Copeman, 'A British Medical Association lecture on immunization against diphtheria, scarlet fever, and measles', *British Medical Journal*, Vol. 1, No. 3515 (19 May 1928), 833–35.
17 'Toxoid and toxin-antitoxin in diphtheria immunization', *British Medical Journal*, Vol. 2, No. 3574 (6 July 1929), 22–23.
18 Anthony Cartwright, 'Medicines regulation', in O'Grady et al, *Medicines, medical devices and the law* (Cambridge, 1999), 25–45.
19 Parish, *Immunization*, 151.
20 Tzen, Dzen and Chang, 'Report on accident following the use of diphtheria toxin-antitoxin mixture', *China Medical Journal*, No. 41 (1927), 412–23.

Australia,[21] and Colombia,[22] influenced the introduction of further regulatory measures in the form of the Therapeutic Substances Regulations 1931. This new legislation sought to ensure the purity, potency, and quality of sera and prophylactics manufactured in Britain, by placing a mandatory obligation on manufacturers to obtain a licence to operate from the Ministry of Health.[23] In addition, the 1931 regulations restricted opportunities to conduct clinical trials in Britain.[24] At Wellcome, Richard O'Brien lamented that these restrictions meant that in England 'the immunologist is always far ahead of the clinical investigator'. He stated:

> When Dr Park in New York wishes to compare the relative values of different methods of immunization – for example, by toxoid given at different doses at different intervals, and with or without the addition of alum – he first investigates the problem, as we do, with laboratory animals, and then repeats the same investigation simultaneously on large groups of comparable children in schools, an opportunity which we in England can regard but with envy.[25]

Despite O'Brien's public rhetoric bemoaning lost opportunities, Wellcome continued to trial experimental anti-diphtheria prophylactics, in a district free of British regulatory restraints.

At the Wellcome Research Laboratory, Alexander Glenny conducted experimental work on the antigenic effects of an alum-toxoid, produced by the addition of aluminium sulphate to a diphtheria toxoid. Glenny's experimental research with guinea pigs conclusively demonstrated that the addition of aluminium sulphate, or potash alum, affected a delayed absorption of toxoid, but also an increased antigenic efficiency. In laboratory trials, Glenny injected 41 guinea pigs with alum-toxoid. Within three weeks, 29 tested Schick negative, and in every case, full immunity developed

---

21 Peter Hobbins, 'Immunization is as popular as a death adder': The Bundaberg tragedy and the politics of medical science in interwar Australia', *Social History of Medicine*, Vol. 24, No. 2 (2011), 426–44.

22 Vincent Manuel Garcia, 'Therapeutic accidents and new health practices. Colombian medicine in the face of the anti-diphtheria vaccination catastrophe of Medellin, 1930', *Historica Crítica*, No. 46, (January/April 2012), 110–31.

23 *The Therapeutic Substance Regulations*, dated 25 July 1931, made by the Joint Committee constituted by sec. 4 (1) of the Acts, S.R. and O. 1931, No. 633.

24 Adrian F. Bristow, et al, 'Standardization of biological medicines: the first hundred years, 1900–2000', *Notes and Records of The Royal Society*, Vol. 60, No. 3 (22 September 2006) 271–89.

25 R. A. O'Brien, 'Immunization in the prevention of specific fevers', *British Medical Journal* (20 October 1934), 712.

within five weeks.[26] Influenced by Glenny's findings, and funded by the American Public Health Association, in the spring of 1931 William Park and May Schroder conducted trials to compare diphtheria toxoid, toxoid plus alum, and toxin-antitoxin on infants and children at the Home for Hebrew Infants, and seven other unidentified institutions in New York.[27] In June 1931, at the international meeting of the Microbiological Society at Paris, Park reported positively on the alum-toxoid trials undertaken in New York. Richard O'Brien, who also attended the Paris conference, informed Park that Wellcome had also trialled experimental alum-toxoid antigens on children, with favourable results.[28] However, Wellcome had not conducted the vaccine trials on British children, but on children in Cork city in the Irish Free State.

Vaccine Trials in Cork City

In November 1930, some six months before Park and Schroder's much celebrated alum-toxoid trials, Jack Saunders conducted a series of Wellcome-sponsored alum-toxoid vaccine trials, involving 436 children, aged eight months to 14 years, in Cork city.[29] Throughout the trials, Saunders maintained contact with Richard O'Brien and Wellcome Research Laboratories, who provided the necessary supply of experimental antigen. Laboratory workers at Wellcome, tasked with the preparation of an antigen with an 'almost complete lack of experience of its use with human beings', are said to have proceeded 'with extreme caution' in regard to the degree of dilution of the toxoid and the proportion of added alum.[30] Four batches of differing toxoid dilution, alum composition, and lethal factor (Lf) values were produced and 'sent gratis' to Saunders; batches B6219 (0.5 per cent alum), B6217 (2.0 per cent alum), B6539 (7.5 per cent alum), and B6707 (9.0 per cent alum).[31]

Although Saunders dispensed with preliminary Schick tests during the trials, a high percentage of children treated with Wellcome's experimental antigens failed to return for a post-treatment test. In order to exercise more control over the trial subjects, and to better assess the efficacy, or

26 A. T. Glenny, 'Insoluble precipitates in diphtheria and tetanus immunization', *British Medical Journal* Vol. 2, (16 August 1930), 244.
27 W. Park and M. Schroder, 'Diphtheria toxin-antitoxin and toxoid; a comparison', *American Journal of Public Health and the Nation's Health*, Vol. 22, No. 1 (January 1932), 7–16. See also, Grodin and Glantz (eds), *Children as research subjects; science, ethics & law* (Oxford, 1994).
28 Park and Schroder, *American Journal of Public Health* (1932), 10.
29 Park and Schroder, *American Journal of Public Health* (1932), 1049.
30 Park and Schroder, *American Journal of Public Health* (1932), 1048.
31 J. C. Saunders, 'Alum-Precipitated Toxoid in diphtheria prevention', *The Lancet*, 1 May 1937, 1064.

otherwise, of Wellcome's antigens, Saunders extended the scope of the trials to include institutional children. Although the institutions involved remain unidentified, Saunders stated that 'there are but two suitable institutions in Cork, both of them orphanages, and they were placed at our disposal by the authorities'.[32]

By April 1931, three distinct groups of children were involved in the Cork trials. The largest group received the TAM antigen while attending the public health clinic and schools. The second group were administered the experimental alum-toxoid antigens, also at the public health clinic and city schools. The third group occupied two orphanages, half of whom received TAM, and half of whom received one of the experimental alum-toxoid antigens. The basis of comparison for the trials fell under three headings: (1) The percentage of negative reactors after immunization in children treated with alum-toxoid and in those treated with toxoid-antitoxin, and the rate of development of immunity in both groups; (2) The number of reported cases of diphtheria occurring in both groups after treatment; (3) The rate of development of immunity in a group of controlled Schick-positive children in institutions.[33]

By the end of 1931, 1,230 children completed the full course of treatment with TAM, and importantly for Saunders, presented for the post-treatment Schick test. The initial Schick test in this group recorded over 80 per cent positive reactors, indicating high susceptibility to diphtheria. When Saunders retested the same group four months after their final inoculation, he found that 75 per cent tested negative: indicating relatively rapid immunity development. Further Schick testing, conducted at monthly intervals, demonstrated that the percentage of negative reactors rose steadily, peaking at 89.5 per cent at the ten-month interval. Taking the group as a whole, post-treatment Schick tests conducted between the four and twelve-month intervals registered an average of 81.2 per cent negative reactors.[34]

At the public health clinic and city schools, 436 children, presented by their parents, were administered Wellcome's experimental alum-toxoid antigens. It is unclear whether Saunders sought parental consent, or if parents were aware that their children were the first human subjects to receive Wellcome's antigens. Henry Parish noted that Saunders insisted that no deviation from the normal intervals of immunization, and dose size of the experimental antigens, should occur, as he feared that any suspicion of 'experimenting' would undermine his campaign. When a health visitor inadvertently mentioned that the public health department were introducing an improved anti-diphtheria preparation,

32 Saunders, 'Alum-Toxoid', *Lancet*, 1932, 1049.
33 Saunders, 'Alum-Toxoid', *Lancet*, 1932, 1049.
34 Saunders, 'Alum-Toxoid', *Lancet*, 1932, 1048.

one mother remarked 'So up to now Dr Saunders has been experimenting'.[35] This astute observation suggests that Saunders failed to obtain informed consent during the Cork vaccine trials.

Therapeutic substance regulations, along the lines of the British model, were not introduced in the Irish Free State until 1932. Vaccine trials undertaken by Saunders during 1930–31 were not subject to any statutory controls relating to the conduct of clinical trials, and with regard to ethical considerations relating to human experimentation; Saunders was governed, to a large degree, by the standards of his time. In the early 1930s, these standards amounted to little more than what David Rothman termed a 'utilitarian ethic' where the benefits to the many which flowed from human experimentation was considered as justification for the lack of a full appreciation of the rights of trial subjects, particularly in regard to obtaining their consent for participation in research.[36] However, the fact that clinical trials undertaken by Saunders went without mention in his annual reports, and that no record of them appears in national or municipal health records suggests that central health, the municipal authority, and the public would not have accepted the highly experimental nature of these trials. Conversely, the most respected British medical journals did publish Saunders's trial findings, which indicates that the Irish and British medical community considered human experimentation, and the manner in which Saunders undertook it, to have been acceptable practice.

Of the 436 children treated with Wellcome's alum-toxoid, 166 failed either to complete treatment or to present for post-treatment Schick testing, suggesting a 'desertion rate' of 38 per cent.[37] In total, 270 children returned for the post-treatment test. Of these, nine received treatment with batch B6219. After an interval of 12 weeks, B6219 achieved a maximum percentage of 66 per cent negative reactors in this group. Among those children who returned for post-treatment testing, 111 received treatment with batch B6217. After an interval of six weeks, B6217 achieved 86.2 per cent negative reactors among this group. A further 62 children treated with batch B6217, and tested at intervals of between seven and 12 weeks, produced 100 per cent negative reactors. Overall, the group treated with batch B6217 produced an average of 95.5 per cent negative reactions.

Also among those who returned were 69 children treated with batch B6539. Of these, 72 retested after an interval of six weeks and 90.2 per cent negative reactors ensued. The remaining 24 children treated with

35 Parish, Notes on visit to Cork.
36 Department of Health, *Report on 3 Clinical Trials involving babies and children in institutional settings 1960/61, 1970 and 1973.*
37 Saunders, *Lancet*, 1932, 1048.

batch B6539 recorded 100 per cent immunity. The remaining 54 returning children received batch B6707. When this group retested more than six weeks after treatment, all gave negative reactions.[38]

Three of the experimental batches, B6217, B6539, and B6707 successfully induced immunity in human subjects within 12 weeks of treatment. These results suggested that Wellcome's alum-toxoid induced rapid immunity and was a substantial improvement over TAM. Furthermore, alum-toxoid achieved 100 per cent negative reactors within twelve weeks, as compared with a maximum 89.5 per cent negative reactors, which took ten months to achieve using TAM.

During 1930, the confirmed post-treatment diphtheria attack rate among Cork children treated with TAM was 2.35 per 1000, as compared with an attack rate of 25.69 per 1000 among untreated children. In the group treated with Wellcome's alum-toxoid, just three post-treatment diphtheria cases occurred. Two cases, a brother and sister, received treatment with batch B6219, a batch found to possess little or no antigenic power, and withdrawn shortly after introduction.[39] The third case, treated with batch B6217, had failed to complete treatment. This boy shared a school desk with a confirmed diphtheria carrier responsible for an acute diphtheria outbreak in which two boys died. Saunders concluded that for practical purposes 'one may reasonably state that there had been no case of post-treatment diphtheria reported among children treated with alum-toxoid'. [40]

In the trial institutions, Saunders found that results obtained utilizing the preliminary Schick tests were 'completely different from those obtained from children generally in the city'. Together, both orphanages presented 405 children, and 38.5 per cent tested Schick positive as compared with 80 per cent of the general child population.[41] Elimination of the unusually high proportion of negative reactors in both institutions reduced the number of children submitted to the final test to 142. Saunders segregated positive reactors into two groups, one treated with TAM, and the other with batch B6539 alum-toxoid.

The first inoculations utilizing alum-toxoid commenced in April 1931 and subsequently at fortnightly intervals. Saunders conceded that the trial

38 Saunders, *Lancet*, 1932, 1048–50.
39 J. C. Saunders, *Trends in diphtheria prophylaxis*, paper read before the Cork Clinical Society, 2 February 1935.
40 Saunders, *Trend of diphtheria prophylaxis*, 119.
41 The high proportion of naturally negative reactors in the Cork city institutions was not unusual. It was estimated by Henry Parish that the natural immunity rate amongst the inmates of the average industrial school or poor-law school in England, was in the region of 60 per cent as compared with over 80 per cent amongst the general population.

sample was much reduced from what he had expected it to be, but asserted that the results were 'sufficiently striking to justify publication [...] as they confirm closely not only our own experience among the child population of the city in general, but also the results obtained by Glenny with guinea pigs'.[42] Post-treatment Schick testing of the institutional children further reflected the relative efficacy of both antigens, and it seems clear that alum-toxoid again proved to be a definite advance on TAM. Saunders's conclusions, based on his experiences treating 436 children with alum-toxoid, and over 7,000 with TAM, successfully confirmed Glenny's observations in human subjects.

In April 1933, just five months after the publication of the Cork vaccine trial findings, Saunders published a follow-on article in the *Lancet* outlining a series of adverse reactions experienced by children in the Cork alum-toxoid trials.[43] Saunders insisted that 'alum-toxoid has proved in my hands a very reliable antigen [...] worth a more extended trial'; however, the appearance of abnormally hard lumps, or indurations, and the formation of abscesses in trial subjects elicited a desire for the 'drawbacks' associated with alum-toxoid 'to be understood as fully as possible'. Saunders observed that the frequency of reactions, or other ill effects, 'bore a definite relationship to the batch of vaccines under review and to the composition of the batch concerned'.[44] For comparison purposes, he adopted the following classification: (1) Slight: cases, which at any time during treatment developed local reaction not exceeding 1 inch in diameter, either with or without slight malaise; (2) Moderate: a local reaction occurring at any time during treatment, extending from 1 to 3 inches in diameter, whether accompanied by pain and malaise or not and (3) Severe: any local reaction exceeding 3 inches in diameter, whether with or without general reaction.

Saunders established that the nine children treated with batch B6219 showed no adverse reactions. Of 132 children treated with batch B6217, eight cases, or 6 per cent experienced reactions mainly of a 'slight' nature. A further four patients, 3 per cent of this group, developed indurations without suffering reactions. Of 150 children treated with batch B6539, 84 cases, or 55.9 per cent of the group, suffered reactions the majority of which were of a 'slight' and 'moderate' nature. Of 220 children treated with batch B6707, 79 cases, or 35.8 per cent of the group, suffered reactions mostly of a 'slight' and 'moderate' nature. However, a considerable increase in the number and proportion of reactions of a 'severe' nature was associated with batch B6707.[45]

42 Saunders, 'Alum-Toxoid', *Lancet*, 1932, 1049.
43 Saunders, 'The reactions with alum-toxoid in diphtheria prophylaxes, *The Lancet*, 15 April 1933, 791–95. See also Saunders, *Trends in diphtheria prophylaxis*, 119.
44 Saunders, 'Reactions with alum-toxoid', *Lancet*, 1933, 791.
45 Saunders, 'Reactions with alum-toxoid', *Lancet*, 1933, 791–92.

Saunders's experience with TAM demonstrated that a reaction to the first injection was a 'fairly reliable index' for any possible subsequent reactions. However, his experience with alum-toxoid showed no regularity in this regard, and in several instances, a reaction occurred only after the third injection. This feature appeared to be 'peculiar to alum-toxoid' and the nature of the reactions showed a direct relationship with the strength of the toxoid, the percentage of alum, and the lethal factor (Lf) value of each batch, although exactly which one was not quite so clear.[46]

Batch B6707 comprised 9 per cent alum, the highest alum content and by far the highest Lf value of the alum-toxoid antigens trialled. Peculiarly, the percentage of adverse reactions recorded for batch B6707 (35.8 per cent) was far lower than those associated with batch B6539 (55.9 per cent), an antigen with a lower 7.56 per cent alum content and a lower lethal factor value than batch B6707. These figures suggest that the antigen responsible for the largest proportion of severe reactions was B6539, the batch used exclusively on institutional children. However, this discrepancy may be more apparent than real. The fact that batch B6539 was used almost exclusively on children in institutions, meant that it was possible for Saunders to maintain effective follow up and to observe reactions that might have otherwise gone unnoticed. All those treated with batch B6707 received treatment at the public health clinic, and of the 436 children presented there, 166 or 38 per cent failed to return for follow-up treatment.[47]

In the regular course of treatment with TAM, a desertion rate of 15 per cent was general. It seems probable that the excess desertion rate (38 per cent) associated with B6707 is attributable to adverse reactions to the first injection; reactions which went undetected due to the number of children who failed to return for the post-treatment test. Considering that B6707 produced most reactions of a 'severe' nature among institutional children, it is highly probable that a sizeable proportion of children who failed to return for retesting at the public health clinic also experienced similarly severe reactions.

Wellcome's batch B6707 proved to be a very efficient antigen in the Cork trials; however, Saunders conceded 'we have experienced more trouble with it than with any other batch we have handled. Reactions have been more pronounced and at one time indurations were a real source of concern'.[48] Although indurations associated with alum-toxoid generally manifest in a slight or transient degree, the periodic occurrence of very marked and semi-permanent indurations had the capacity to act as a deterrent to the widespread adoption of alum-toxoid. Saunders followed up

46 Saunders, 'Reactions', *Lancet*, 1933, 791.
47 Saunders, 'Alum-Toxoid', *Lancet*, 1932, 1048.
48 Saunders, 'Reactions with alum-toxoid', *Lancet*, 1933, 792.

all recorded instances of indurations with a personal examination of each case to determine if the varying degrees of indurations were of a permanent character. For comparative purposes, he adopted the following standards: (1) Slight: transient thickening and hardening of the subcutaneous tissues about the size of a pea; (2) Moderate: as above, but attaining approximately to the size of a broad bean; (3) Marked: as above, but attaining to the size of a florin piece or more or any induration lasting more than two months and including all cases in which there has been abscess formation.[49]

The nine children treated with B6219, suffered no indurations. Of 132 children treated with B6217, four developed 'mild' indurations. On re-examination, two years after treatment, no trace of 'hardening' and no 'history of trouble' afflicted this group. Of 150 children treated with B6539, three developed 'definitely established' indurations. After a period of eighteen months, these children were reportedly 'in excellent health'. Saunders examined every institutional child, also after eighteen months, and none suffered an induration. With regard to B6707, Saunders conceded that this batch had 'caused more trouble with induration than any of the others that we have tried'. Of 220 children treated with B6707, 33 developed indurations. Of these, 18 were 'mild' cases, six were 'moderate' and the remaining nine cases presented with 'marked' indurations.[50]

The whole question of the suitability of alum-toxoid as a diphtheria prophylactic hinged around these 'marked cases' and as Saunders regarded them as being 'of the greatest importance', he discussed them individually. The affected children ranged in age from 15 months to ten years, and all received treatment at the public health immunization clinic on dates between 11 June and 8 October 1931. In every case, children suffered 'unduly long and persistent induration' lasting between 13 and 17 months. The experience of one ten-year-old boy designated C. D. played out thus:

After second dose of AMT (alum-toxoid), developed a very marked inflammatory reaction extending practically from shoulder to elbow. Gradually subsided to an area of 2.5 square inches, over which inflammation persisted for some time longer and which appeared at one time to be going to abscess formation. Eventually cleared up completely.
Sept. 25th: Schick test negative. Some redness still present over back of left arm. No pain or tenderness.
Dec. 7th, 1932: No trace of induration. Arm quite normal in all respects. General health excellent.[51]

49 Saunders, 'Reactions', *Lancet*, 1933, 792–93.
50 Saunders, *Lancet*, 1933, 793.
51 Saunders, *Lancet*, 1933, 793.

The majority of cases resolved themselves in this fashion. However, four children experienced abscess formation as a sequel to induration. In these instances, children developed a localized abscess on the arm at the site of injection. In every case, the abscess discharged for a while, and then healed completely leaving a small scar.[52]

In spite of the adverse reactions, Saunders concluded that he was 'quite satisfied' with the results obtained by the application of Wellcome's alum-toxoid antigens, and in particular 'the immunising efficiency of the product'.[53] News of adverse reactions caused some concerns at Wellcome. Richard O'Brien, in particular, was not satisfied that the company had produced a vaccine suitable for general release, and he informed Saunders that Wellcome had decided on a 'temporary suspension of supplies'.[54]

Following the withdrawal of Wellcome's alum-toxoid antigens, Richard O'Brien issued Saunders with another new prophylactic Formol Toxoid (FT). Originally developed by Gaston Ramon in France, Charles Pope produced a more potent toxin through an improved method of cultivating the diphtheria organism. Saunders introduced FT in Cork in mid-1933, and deemed it 'a great improvement on TAM'. A full course of treatment with FT involved just two injections. This reduced the mandatory number of attendances at the public health clinic, and eased administrative work considerably.[55] However, FT had a liability to elicit adverse reactions, particularly in older children. Contemporary accepted teaching stressed that the administration of FT to children aged eight years and older, without undertaking a preliminary Moloney Test[56] to detect possible reactors, was unsafe practice.[57] Likely reactors to the FT antigen were, as a rule, administered TAF as a safer, albeit more expensive, alternative. During 1933 and 1934, Saunders administered FT to 1,716 children in Cork city; however, the results of Saunders's intervention with FT remain unpublished.[58]

52 Saunders, 'Reactions with alum-toxoid', *Lancet*, 1933, 794.
53 J. C. Saunders, 'Alum-precipitated toxoid in diphtheria prevention', *Lancet*, 1 May 1937, 1064–68.
54 J. C. Saunders, *Lancet*, 1 May 1937, 1064–68.
55 J. C. Saunders, *Report of the Chief Medical Officer of Health for 1934* (Eagle Printing, Cork, 1935), 29.
56 The 'Moloney Test' is a diphtheria toxoid-reaction test introduced in Toronto during 1927 by P. J. Moloney and C. J. Fraser for detecting individuals likely to have an undesirable reaction to the administration of diphtheria toxoid. See E. Ashworth Underwood, 'The diphtheria toxoid-reaction (Moloney) test: its applications and significance', *Journal of Hygiene* (London), Vol. 35, No. 4, (December 1935), 449–75 and Robert Sawyer, 'Diphtheria formol toxoid and the Moloney test', *The Lancet*, Vol. 226, No. 5836 (6 July 1935), 22.
57 Saunders, *Trends in diphtheria prophylaxis*, 120.
58 Saunders, *Report 1934*, 24.

Further Vaccine Trials

In 1934, Wellcome issued a purified batch of FT antigen to Dr Christopher McSweeney, Superintendent of the City Isolation Hospital, Canton, Cardiff. McSweeney, a Corkonian and one-time classmate of Jack Saunders, reported that this batch of FT 'showed no improvement' on the batch used by Saunders in Cork.[59] While McSweeney expressed satisfaction with the efficacy of Wellcome's FT antigen, he cautioned that 'this particular prophylactic is not yet on the market' and was obtained from Richard O'Brien 'for experimental purposes only'.[60] FT, and its diluted derivative MT, found few advocates in Britain or Ireland as associated adverse reactions precluded them from commercial use.

McSweeney, followed Saunders's work with alum-toxoid with some interest, and hailed him to be the first European field immunologist to 'try the experimental antigen on a large scale'. However, McSweeney observed that the 'great many reactions, not a few of them severe had dashed any hopes which would have been entertained in respect of alum preparations in the home countries'. He noted that some batches of Wellcome's alum-toxoid supplied to Saunders contained 9 per cent alum, and opined that the resultant severe reactions 'though unfortunate, can hardly be wondered at'.[61]

At Wellcome, Richard O'Brien and his colleagues contemplated how the 'troublesome local reaction' produced by alum-toxoid could be circumvented. In America, Wells, Graham, and Havens successfully modified Glenny and Barr's' alum-toxoid formula to produce an antigen of low alum content. Despite some guinea pig fatalities due to pneumonia, clinical trials of this new 'single shot' alum precipitate antigen (APT) extended to include children in New York institutions.[62] The published results showed that the modified formula had high potency, was quick acting, and demonstrated 'a complete absence of severe reactions'. At Wellcome, Richard O'Brien secured samples of the modified antigen from his American colleagues. Having conducted laboratory-based tests; O'Brien concluded that 'persistent lumps and rare sterile abscesses still disturb the picture' and that the American preparations 'did not provide better results than our own'.[63] Under O'Brien's

59 Parish, *Immunization*, 149.
60 C. J. McSweeney, 'The prevention of diphtheria', *Irish Journal of Medical Science*, Vol. 10, No. 2 (February 1935), 76–81.
61 McSweeney, 'The prevention of diphtheria', 80.
62 Wells, D. M., Graham, H. and Havens, L. C., 'Diphtheria toxoid precipitated with alum: its preparation and advantages', *American Journal of Public Health*, Vol. 22, No. 6 (June 1932), 648–50.
63 R. A. O'Brien, 'Immunization in the prevention of specific fevers', *British Medical Journal* (20 October 1934), 712–14.

direction, Charles Pope produced modified versions of the Glenny and Barr APT formula in pursuit of what Wellcome perceived as 'the preparation of an ideal precipitate': an antigen composed of minimal alum content and maximum toxoid content.[64] Wellcome's laboratory-based experiments achieved the desired result, but British legislation continued to prohibit a progression to clinical trials on human subjects. That his American counterparts had opportunities available to trial new vaccines in human subjects was a state of affairs which O'Brien lamented: 'we in England can only regard but with envy'. While O'Brien publicly bemoaned the lack of opportunities to conduct clinical trials of Wellcome's modified alum-toxoid in Britain, privately he explored his options.

In February 1934, Wellcome dispatched a batch of modified APT to Christopher McSweeney in Cardiff. In a private correspondence O'Brien apologized to McSweeney 'for plaguing you with too many suggestion' but reasoned that:

The number of people with clinical opportunities and the time and keenness to carry out much-needed observations of this kind is very small. They are indeed a 'select band'.[65]

Prompted by advances reported in American scientific literature, McSweeney agreed to undertake trials to compare two of Wellcome's experimental anti-diphtheria antigens, FT and APT. McSweeney asserted that the experiments were rendered possible only by the 'courtesy and kindness' of Richard O'Brien of the Wellcome Research Laboratories, 'who supplied the whole of the materials with which it was carried out'.[66] In February 1934, O'Brien notified McSweeney that Wellcome had a new batch of alum-toxoid ready. However, he cautioned:

On animals, it is apparently innocuous. We do not know anything about its effects on humans [...] I would suggest that you use on the first few children only a small dose [...] If you would like to have some of the batch I could supply you with a reasonable number of doses from our stock free of charge.[67]

64 O'Brien, 'Immunization', *British Medical Journal* (1934), 712.
65 Letter from Richard O'Brien to Christopher McSweeney, 22 December 1933, Royal College of Physicians Ireland, Cork Street Fever Hospital and Cherry Orchard Hospital Papers, CSFH/3/1/2/7.
66 C. J. McSweeney, 'An evaluation of modern diphtheria prophylactics', *British Medical Journal* (19 January 1935), 103–05.
67 Letter from Richard O'Brien to Christopher McSweeney, 19 February 1934, Royal College of Physicians Ireland (RCPI), *Cork Street Fever Hospital and Cherry Orchard Hospital Papers*, CSFH/3/1/2/7.

Regarding the clinical subjects, McSweeney stated:

> The experimental material was drawn from two residential institutions
> (contributing respectively 109 and 213 children), nine smaller homes
> (ninety-eight children), a hospital for rheumatic children (fourteen
> children), and two elementary schools (185 children), while twenty-
> three children convalescent from scarlet fever or measles were also
> included, giving a total of 642 children.[68]

Preliminary Schick tests in the Cardiff institutions showed that 424 of 642
children originally selected for the trials tested Schick negative. McSweeney
noted, that while 'these institutions were particularly suitable' for controlled
experiments, he expressed 'disappointment' that so many institutional
children returned negative Schick results, necessitating their exclusion from
the trials. A second complication, which further attenuated the original
control group, was that the Moloney Test identified a significant number of
children demonstrating high sensitivity to the FT antigen. While McSweeney
did not eliminate these children from the investigation, he did adhere to
contemporary best practice and administered TAF to this group. Although
203 children were subsequently involved in the Cardiff trials, McSweeney
noted that 'due to a variety of unavoidable causes', only 187 completed the
full course of treatment. In February 1934, McSweeney administered the
experimental APT vaccine (Serial No. B8725) to 78 children. He resolved to
administer the first injections cautiously: these were the first human subjects
to receive it. The first group, comprising 21 children, received 0.1 c.cm of
APT and in those showing no adverse reaction dosage steadily increased to
0.25 c.cm, 0.65 c.cm and 1.0 c.cm, administered at fortnightly intervals. As
McSweeney gained more experience with batch B8725, the initial dosage
increased to 0.5 c.cm, and subsequently to 1.0 c.cm. No child received more
than 2.0 c.cm of APT in total. Every child received a posterior Schick test
four weeks after treatment.[69]

A second group, comprising 86 children, received two 1.0 c.cm shots of
potent FT (Serial No. B8553), administered at fortnightly intervals. Children
who showed a local reaction to the initial injection received the second dose
in two instalments of 0.5 c.cm over two successive weeks. The final group
comprised 39 children, all of whom registered Schick positive/Moloney
positive reactions. This group were unsuitable candidates for FT or APT
and received three 1.0 c.cm injections of TAF.[70] McSweeney's analysis of the

68 McSweeney, *British Medical Journal* (1935), 103.
69 McSweeney, *British Medical Journal* (1935), 103.
70 McSweeney, *British Medical Journal* (1935), 104.

efficacy of Wellcome's anti-diphtheria prophylactics reveals that the potent FT antigen produced the best results, inducing immunity in 88.1 per cent of children after four weeks. TAF produced the next best set of results inducing immunity in 83.3 per cent of children after four weeks. However, the results achieved using APT were much less satisfactory, inducing immunity in just 77.3 per cent of children over the equivalent period.

Although no general reactions occurred, 58.8 per cent of those treated with APT suffered some form of local reaction, almost three times the rate associated with FT and TAF. While McSweeney encountered no abscess formation, he noted that local reactions associated with APT occurred 'in varying degrees of intensity mainly consisting of areas of erythema varying from one to four inches in diameter'. Considering that these reactions to APT occurred in Moloney negative children, it must be reasonable to suggest that APT would have induced increased and more severe adverse reactions among the general child population. Notwithstanding, 75 out of a possible 78 children, or 96 per cent of those treated with APT, completed treatment and returned for the post-treatment Schick test. This suggests that severe reactions were not associated with this particular batch of APT. Seven children who suffered local reactions following the first dose of APT subsequently received two shots of TAF; another indication that reactions were not so severe as to act as a deterrent to return for further treatment.[71]

Of those children administered FT, 21.5 per cent experienced local reactions. Among this group, 76 out of a possible 86 children completed the full course of treatment and returned for retesting four weeks after treatment. The 12 per cent desertion rate among this group suggests that FT caused adverse reactions severe enough to deter a substantial proportion from completing treatment. Although 4 per cent of children administered APT also failed to complete the full course of treatment, the substantially higher desertion rate among children treated with FT suggests that reactions to this antigen were of greater severity.

The Cardiff trials demonstrated that, in terms of rapidity and efficacy, Wellcome's anti-diphtheria antigens APT, FT, and TAF were a definite advance on TAM. However, APT was prone to induce local reactions, which militated against its use among the general population. The general advantages seemed to lie with FT, however, the associated requirement for a preliminary Moloney test necessitated an extra intradermal injection, and by extension, an extra visit for inspection purposes. This impracticality ruled out FT for general use.

On Richard O'Brien's recommendation, McSweeney trialled a 'universal' or 'detector dose' of FT on a group of children without performing a

71 McSweeney, 'Immunization', *British Medical Journal* (1935), 104.

preliminary Moloney test.[72] O'Brien reasoned that a minute dose would cause a slight reaction in FT sensitive children. If this proved to be the case, then the Moloney test would be redundant. McSweeney administered a minute dose of FT to 18 children: five immediately showed 'marked local reactions' and a further two experienced local reactions. McSweeney concluded that FT was a highly efficient antigen, but that it is was ideally suited to use in the controlled environment of residential institutions only. McSweeney was less impressed with Wellcome's APT antigen. He concluded that APT had not compared favourably with either FT or TAF, and that its tendency to produce local redness was 'a contraindication to its general use outside institutions'.[73] O'Brien was deeply disappointed with McSweeney's findings and remonstrated, regarding APT, that Burroughs Wellcome had been placed in 'a very unfair commercial position' compared with their American competitors. O'Brien claimed that despite 'clear evidence of haste and hurry in the American literature', American-produced APT antigens were being sold in large quantities throughout Britain.[74] Despite O'Brien's concerns and McSweeney's reservations, Wellcome's experimental APT antigen again found its way to Jack Saunders in Cork city.

Saunders's experience as a field immunologist taught him that any method involving multiple injections would not induce complete communal immunity: 'considerable leakage' or 'considerable desertion' was to be expected. In previous years, up to 32 per cent of children failed to complete treatment, which Saunders attributed to 'the objection inherent in so many people to hypodermic injections'. He contended that any scheme characterized by such high desertion rates must be 'written down as a failure', remedied by reducing injections to the minimum, without inducing a reduction in the degree of protection conferred.[75] The great virtue claimed by Wellcome's 'one-shot' APT antigen was that it would protect children with a single injection. Saunders concluded that if substantiated, this would constitute an important immunological breakthrough.

In December 1934, Wellcome's modified alum-toxoid, APT, arrived in Cork city. In his annual report, Saunders stated that APT was 'no novelty' to the people of Cork, a city that could claim to be 'one of the pioneer cities so far as the use of alum-toxoid is concerned'.[76] He noted that 'the suspension and further investigation' of the APT antigen culminated in a 'very much

72 R. A. O'Brien, 'Diphtheria prophylaxes', *British Medical Journal* (2 February 1935), 232.
73 McSweeney, 'Immunization', *British Medical Journal* (1935), 105.
74 Letter from Richard O'Brien to Christopher McSweeney, 4 February 1935, RCPI, Cork Street Fever Hospital and Cherry Orchard Hospital Papers, CSFH/3/1/2/7.
75 Saunders, 'Alum precipitated toxoid', *Lancet*, 1937, 1064.
76 Saunders, *Report 1934*, 30.

improved article, which appears to have achieved the ideal; protection with one injection'.

Between December 1934 and December 1936, Saunders administered APT to 2,791 children, 250 of whom resided in a residential institution for boys.[77] To keep the number of injections to a minimum, he dispensed with the preliminary Schick test in children aged seven years and under. This group initially received 1 c.cm. APT and instructions to re-attend for a Schick test after five weeks. Children aged seven years and older were subjected to concurrent Schick and Moloney tests on their first visits.

As adverse reactions generally occurred in children aged seven years or older, Saunders employed the Moloney test among this age group to indicate any possible negative reaction.[78] If a child recorded an initial Schick negative reaction, no further treatment ensued. If a child recorded a Schick positive/Moloney negative result, treatment with APT followed. In cases where a child recorded a Schick positive/Moloney positive result, Saunders abandoned APT in favour of the safer alternative TAF.

After a relatively short retesting interval of just five weeks, 99.0 per cent of children treated with APT had developed full immunity. Previous immunization rates, recorded in association with the use of TAM, produced a maximum rate of 89.5 per cent: achieved after a greatly extended interval of ten months. The administration of potent FT during 1933–34 secured a maximum immunization rate of 96.8 per cent and required two injections. Although Saunders achieved similarly high immunization rates with earlier batches of alum-toxoid, this required multiple injections and adverse reactions ensued. Saunders concluded that Wellcome's 'single shot' APT antigen was 'very effective as an immunising agent' and that 'it remains to be seen how the results obtained compared with those in other places'.[79] While Isabolinski, Judenitsch, and Lewzow (1935), Kositza (1935), Schmidt-Burbach (1936), and Faragó (1935) also trialled APT, Saunders's work was the only research involving human experimentation. In every other case, experiments involved laboratory animals only.

Not all observers valued Wellcome's APT. However, Saunders resolved that those with 'considerable experience of APT in actual field work' would continue to use it 'among suitable groups of children'.[80] Wellcome's APT certainly demonstrated an unsurpassed efficacy and potency, and numbers of non-returnees, or desertions, were negligible. The added bonus, as the

77 Saunders, *Report 1936*, 17.
78 C. J. McSweeney, 'The prevention of diphtheria', paper read before the Medical Society, University College Dublin, on 3 December 1934.
79 Saunders, 'Alum precipitated toxoid', *Lancet*, 1937, 1065.
80 Saunders, 'Alum precipitated toxoid', *Lancet*, 1937, 1066.

American trials confirmed, was that adverse reactions associated with this antigen were, 'definitely less than with the older batches', particularly in relation to abscess formation.

Saunders cautioned parents to report to the public health clinic if they experienced any anxiety in relation to their children developing sore arms, or indeed, if any post-treatment general sickness ensued. Very few subsequently did so. Although 'a very large proportion' of parents were 'quite emphatic' that no adverse reactions occurred, post-treatment check-ups found that 313 children experienced some form of adverse reaction. Over 6.0 per cent of children aged less than 2 years experienced a mild reaction, however, reactions were more frequent and more severe among older children. Among eight to ten year-olds, 45.4 per cent experienced some reaction, one in three being of a severe type.[81] Although no abscess formation occurred, every child developed some form of post-treatment induration. Saunders asserted these were 'of a non-permanent nature and disappeared soon after treatment'. In this respect also, Saunders concluded that Wellcome's APT was a vast improvement on earlier batches.

The introduction of APT to Cork corresponded with an almost simultaneous decline in diphtheria morbidity. While the introduction of TAM in 1929 and the subsequent introduction of alum-toxoid early in 1931 induced a considerable abatement in the severity of the diphtheria epidemic, a more pronounced decline was associated with the rollout of APT in 1935. Wellcome's single shot APT antigen facilitated the treatment of a large number of pre-school children, and proved to be a useful tool in addressing the 'almost insuperable hindrance to mass immunization': that being, the large numbers of children who failed to present for more than one injection.[82]

In Dublin, an immunization scheme exclusively focused on pre-school children largely failed to persuade parents to present children for treatment. Although the susceptible child population of the city numbered 122,000, by 1935 little more than 14,800 children presented for treatment, 1,822 of whom failed to complete the full course.[83] The Dublin scheme, conducted by Dr Denis Hanley, under the supervision of chief medical officer, Matt Russell, sought to negate the necessity to implement immunization schemes in city schools by supplying them with already protected children. However, this limited scheme met with limited success. Rising diphtheria morbidity combined with a high attack rate among children aged 5–9 years highlighted the vulnerability of children of school-going age.

81 Saunders, *Lancet*, 1937, 1067.
82 Saunders, 'Alum precipitated toxoid', *Lancet*, 1937, 1067.
83 D. F. Hanley, 'Anti-diphtheria immunization', *Irish Journal of Medical Science*, Vol. 12, No. 9 (1937), 578–85.

From November 1934 to January 1935, the public health department visited eleven schools with a combined total of 8,817 students. While students reportedly 'presented themselves willingly for the first injection', each successive visit met with increasing reluctance to submit for treatment, and coincided with a 'definite drop in school attendance'. Frustrated with the rate of progress, and inspired by Saunders's success in Cork city, Hanley decided to explore the possibility of substituting the three-shot TAM antigen with Wellcome's, still experimental, one-shot APT. For Hanley, a one-shot antigen would reduce the number of defaulters, expedite the work and reduce any interruption of school routine.[84]

In Dublin, written parental consent was mandatory before subjecting a child to immunization treatment. Hanley attests that of 8,817 students attending the three city schools visited, 54 per cent of parents (4,799) returned consent forms.[85] Interestingly, Saunders's extensive literature on the Cork trials never mentioned the issue of informed consent. Although Hanley secured parental consent, it is unlikely that parents in Dublin or Cork were aware that their children were administered highly experimental material.

Owing to the varied reports in relation to the suitability and efficacy of APT, Hanley opted to undertake 'experimental tests' to establish whether APT was a suitable substance for use on a wide scale in Dublin. With the 'consent and co-operation' of the medical superintendent and staff of the South Dublin Union, Hanley administered APT to 24 institutional children, varying in age from seven months to 14 years. Satisfied that the trial had not produced 'an unduly high percentage' of reactions Hanley took further steps to ascertain the immunizing power of the substance.[86]

Early in 1935, Hanley sought, and was 'readily granted', permission to test APT from the authorities at three children's residential institutions: St Vincent's Industrial School, Goldenbridge, St Joseph's Institute for Deaf and Dumb Boys, Cabra, and St Saviours Orphanage, Lower Dominick Street, Dublin. A combined 360 children, varying in age from four to 15 years were Schick tested, and Hanley deemed the results as both 'surprising' and 'shocking'. As Saunders and McSweeney previously discovered, institutional children recorded much greater rates of natural

---

84 Hanley, 'Anti-diphtheria immunization', *Irish Journal of Medical Science*, 581. A letter from Richard O'Brien to Christopher McSweeney on 4 February 1935 confirms that Wellcome's APT antigen was not available commercially. RCPI, Cork Street Fever Hospital and Cherry Orchard Hospital Papers, CSFH/3/1/2/7.

85 On average, 54 per cent written parental consents were procured. St Vincent de Paul School, Marino provided the highest proportion of consents (71 per cent), and the Meath Street National School provided the least (40 per cent).

86 Hanley, 'Anti-diphtheria immunization', *Irish Journal of Medical Science*, 581.

immunity, and children in the Dublin institutions were no different. Of the 360 children tested, 314 returned a negative Schick reaction and were excluded from further tests.

Hanley administered APT to the remaining 46 children. He monitored them for two weeks after treatment and concluded that 'in no case was there evidence of reactions, local or general'. Indurations 'about the size of a pea' occurred in every case but absorbed gradually. The post-treatment test revealed that 45 children converted to produce a Schick negative reaction: the results confirmed by blood tests undertaken by Richard O'Brien at Wellcome. Emboldened by the results of his own investigation, Hanley recommended the introduction of APT to replace TAM as the main immunizing agent in Dublin city schools and the pre-school clinics.

Between February and October 1935, Hanley administered still experimental APT to 39,267 schoolchildren. He liaised with teachers and parents urging them to report any post-treatment abnormalities. Although 89 children subsequently reported adverse reactions Hanley conceded that there may have been many others that went unreported. Reactions took the form of local inflammation at the site of inoculation, cold abscesses, general reactions accompanied by headache and a high temperature, and some children developed a marked inflammation extending from shoulder to wrist. In every case, children returned to good health after three or four days, and Hanley was satisfied that with regard to the large number of children treated, the number of reactions noted was 'exceedingly small'.[87]

The widespread adoption of APT in Dublin did elicit some negative results. Wellcome's TAM antigen drew criticism because of the high incidence of post-treatment diphtheria associated with it, though the large-scale Dublin campaign showed that APT proved no better in this regard. Of 12,980 children treated with TAM, 27 children, or 0.2 per cent subsequently contracted diphtheria. Of 39,267 children treated with APT, 75 children, or 0.19 per cent subsequently contracted diphtheria. Although Saunders asserted that no post-treatment cases of diphtheria were associated with the use of APT in Cork, it seems clear from the Dublin records that in this regard, APT was no improvement on TAM.[88]

A more worrying outcome of the Dublin APT campaign was that seven post-treatment diphtheria fatalities occurred. One case, a nine-year-old child, received only one injection of TAF, and remained susceptible to the disease. Among the other fatalities, five children received treatment with APT, and one child received full treatment with TAM. In essence, 80 per cent of post-treatment diphtheria fatalities in Dublin occurred in children treated

87 Hanley, 'Anti-diphtheria immunization', *Irish Journal of Medical Science*, 584–85.
88 Saunders, *Trend of diphtheria prophylaxis*, 119.

with Wellcome's 'one-shot' APT antigen, which failed to convey immunity, or it seems any level of protection against the disease to these unfortunate children. These figures stand in sharp contrast with Saunders's findings, who insisted that while some children treated with APT did develop a mild post-treatment diphtheria infection, no fatality had ensued.[89]

In 1935, medical officers trialled Wellcome's APT antigen in children's residential institutions in Tipperary. An article in the *British Medical Journal*, authored by Dr M. Naughten, medical officer of health for County Tipperary South Riding, Dr J. H. White, and Dr A. Foley related to APT 'in respect to its effects on a number of children on whom it was tried out'.[90] They stated 'the material for the investigation consisted of 370 children in three residential institutions'. Although the institutions are not identified it seems reasonable to suggest that the trials were conducted at St Bernard's Industrial School, Fethard, St Francis's Industrial School, Cashel, and St Joseph's Industrial School Clonmel, as these were the only children's residential institutions in Tipperary South.

In this instance, the scope of the trials was limited to children aged ten years and older. Initial Schick Tests revealed 'an unusually high percentage of positive reactors' (ranging between 30 per cent and 53 per cent) all of whom were administered 1 c.cm of APT by deep subcutaneous injection without the application of a Moloney test. Mirroring results recorded in Cork and Dublin, the Tipperary trials also demonstrated the high immunogenic properties of APT, which converted 94 per cent of positive reactors to negative less than eight weeks after treatment. However, the issue of adverse reactions appears to have remained unresolved.

The reactions encountered in Tipperary fell into four groups. The most common and 'almost universal' reaction took the form of 'a small painless induration' at the site of injection. The second affected 10 per cent of treated children and took the form of 'a diffuse erythema' extending around an area of three inches from the site of injection. The third type appeared as 'a brawny induration with hyperaemia' covering the whole arm accompanied by stiffness in the joints and local heat, affecting six children. In one case, 'a minute sterile abscess' appeared at the puncture site. Minor reactions did not alarm Naughten et al; however, they concluded that if the reactions could be rendered less severe without impairing efficiency 'we believe that we would be in possession of an ideal agent for immunization'. Furthermore, Doctors Naughten, White, and Foley were so impressed with

89 J. C. Saunders, 'The occurrence of diphtheria in "immunised" persons', *Irish Journal of Medical Science*, Vol. 8, No. 11 (November 1933), 611–19.

90 Naughten, White, Foley, 'Prevention of diphtheria by the "one-shot" method using alum-precipitated toxoid', *British Medical Journal* (9 November 1935), 893.

the efficacy of Wellcome's APT that they expressed 'a desire to carry out large-scale campaigns in other districts using the same material'.[91]

The published results of the Irish APT vaccine trials elicited a strong desire among many British medical officers to try out the new 'potent diphtheria prophylactics' for themselves.[92] A plethora of articles and correspondences in the British Medical Journal during 1935 and 1936 suggests that many British medical officers had undertaken evaluations of Wellcome's APT prophylactic themselves, and calls for a government backed anti-diphtheria immunization scheme utilizing APT lay at the heart of a burgeoning immunization debate.[93] One correspondent, Dr Guy Bousfield, director of the public health laboratory at Camberwell, South London, claimed that British interest in the APT antigen had increased to the extent that he had been inundated with inquiries 'as to the advisability of "one-shot" active immunization against diphtheria'. Bousfield asserted that 'a determined effort was being made to persuade local authorities and general practitioners to adopt the one-shot method', although he did not elaborate on the source of that pressure. In the face of overwhelmingly positive reaction to the Irish APT trials among British public health doctors, a dissenting Bousfield cautioned:

'One-shot' immunization is ahead of its time. We who have been working for many years have achieved success by careful and thorough work, and now that a considerable section of the public have become converted to the idea of immunization it behoves beginners to refrain from upsetting the apple-cart.[94]

Bousfield's warning proved to be a self-fulfilling prophecy. In November 1936, a routine anti-diphtheria immunization scheme undertaken in County Waterford resulted in 24 children contracting tuberculosis, and the death of a 12-year-old girl.

---

91 Naughten, et al, British Medical Journal (1935), 893.
92 E. Ashford Underwood, "One-shot' Immunization against diphtheria, British Medical Journal (23 June 1934), 1140.
93 Underwood, British Medical Journal (June 1934), 1140; 'Diphtheria immunization', BMJ (16 June 1934), 1081–82; Guy Bousfield, 'Diphtheria Immunization', BMJ (26 January 1935), 181; 'Immunization against diphtheria', BMJ (9 November 1935), 908–09; 'Diphtheria prophylactic APT', BMJ (2 March 1935), 420; George Chesney, 'Alum-precipitated Toxoid in diphtheria immunization', BMJ (1 February 1936), 208–9; H. J. Parish, 'Immunization against diphtheria with Alum-Precipitated Toxoid (APT)', BMJ (1 February 1936), 209–10.
94 Bousfield, 'Diphtheria immunization', British Medical Journal (1935), 181.

Chapter 5
The Ring College Immunization Disaster

In September 1935, Dr Michael O'Farrell, Waterford CMO, put forward a proposal to introduce anti-diphtheria immunization in the county. The board of health sanctioned the scheme, and ordered 144 25 c.c. bottles of TAF antigen from Burroughs Wellcome, Beckenham, Kent, through the Dublin based medical suppliers, Fannin & Company.[1] Over the course of twelve months, 1,070 children received 3,378 injections of TAF without incident.[2] In September 1936, following representations by the local government department, O'Farrell encouraged school principals in Dungarvan to implement anti-diphtheria immunization schemes. The administrators of St Augustine's Friary School in Dungarvan and Ring College, a private boarding school located outside the town, secured parental permission to have their students treated and authorized Dr Daniel McCarthy[3] to proceed with inoculations at both schools.[4] McCarthy secured ten bottles of Wellcome's toxin TAF antigen from O'Farrell's local government stock, and commenced immunization at St Augustine's and at Ring College.[5]

McCarthy visited St Augustine's over the course of three days in November 1936, where he treated 44 children with parental consent. On three separate days, McCarthy treated 38 children, including two of his own, at Ring College.[6] Each child received three 1 c.c shots at weekly intervals, and following standard 'three-shot' procedure, children received the first and third injections in the right arm, and the second injection in the left arm.[7] No complications ensued and in due course, the children returned home for the Christmas holidays.

1 *Irish Times*, 7 February 1939.
2 *Irish Times*, 12 June 1937.
3 *Dungarvan Observer*, 22 May 1937.
4 *Irish Times*, 7 May 1939.
5 WA/PRL/HP/Sub/33/5. Daniel McCarthy, Report on diphtheria immunization in Ring College, 23 February 1937.
6 *Irish Times*, 20 May 1937.
7 R. P. McDonnell, Note on Dungarvan outbreak, 1.

In early January 1937, McCarthy received a visit from Bríd Bean Uí Cionnfaola, mother of Siobhán O'Cionnfaola, a 12-year-old girl who received immunization treatment at Ring College, stating that her daughter was suffering from a sore arm, which developed during the Christmas holidays.[8] On examination, McCarthy found Siobhán to be in poor health, anaemic, and debilitated. Furthermore, the girl's axillary glands were enlarged and tender, and a small discharging ulcer had developed on her right arm, where she received the intramuscular injection. McCarthy advised Bean Uí Cionnfaola regarding treatment of the local condition and prescribed for her daughter's general health.[9]

In early February 1937, Jack Saunders, Cork city's chief medical officer, learned that two children were under private medical care in Cork city following immunization treatment at Ring College. Both children complained of sore arms during the Christmas holidays, but the matter escaped close attention until Christmas Day when their mother, Mrs Cussen, became alarmed and summoned a doctor. The attending physician, Dr Carney, observed that both children had enlarged axillary glands, and he found it necessary to open abscesses to let out 'a good table spoon of pus'. Severe reactions and abscess formation were common following intramuscular injections, but in this case, Carney noted signs of infection generally only found in tubercular patients. He sought a second opinion.[10]

Jack Saunders was a highly experienced immunologist, and widely regarded as the foremost authority on anti-diphtheria immunization in the Free State. On Carney's request, Saunders saw the children and became 'immediately alarmed'. As a field immunologist, he had administered anti-diphtheria serum to over 29,000 children; however, the Cussen children presented an appearance that he had never seen in any immunization case. The children suffered chronic oedema, discharging bruises, diffuse indurations, and enlarged axillary glands. An anxious and increasingly fearful Mrs Cussen, showed Saunders a letter from Ring College headmaster, Séamus 'An Fear Mór' Ó hEocha, confirming that another 'sixteen or seventeen children' treated at his school were similarly affected.[11]

These developments caused Saunders some concern. He pioneered anti-diphtheria immunization in the Irish Free State for close to eight years, and under his supervision Cork city received international recognition as 'the most immunised city in Europe'.[12] Furthermore, Saunders used

8 *Dungarvan Observer*, 22 May 1937.
9 *Irish Times*, 20 May 1937.
10 WA/PRL/HP/Sub/33/5. J. C. Saunders, Letter to R. A. O'Brien, 23 February 1937.
11 Saunders, Letter to R. A. O'Brien, 23 February 1937.
12 John McLeod, *Proceedings of the Royal Society of Medicine*, July 1936, Vol. XXIX (Section on pathology).

anti-diphtheria prophylactics manufactured by Burroughs Wellcome exclusively, the same company who supplied the antigen used at Ring. Notwithstanding his concern for the affected children, Saunders realized that if Mrs Cussen's assertions were indeed true, the negative impact on future immunization schemes would be profound. However, it was three months since McCarthy undertook the inoculations at Ring College and Saunders thought it strange that such a serious incident had not become public.

Saunders wrote to Michael O'Farrell in Waterford, to put the facts of the case before him. A subsequent conversation with 'a practicing surgeon', and county pathologist Dr William O'Donovan of University College, Cork, eased Saunders's suspicion of the presence of tuberculosis in the afflicted children. He could not, however, explain what he had seen, and had been told about the other cases. Commenting on the case, O'Donovan remarked that if Saunders's story should prove to be true, then they could be dealing with a 'second Lübeck'.[13] O'Donovan's reference to the Lübeck disaster is noteworthy. In that instance, a German laboratory mistakenly issued a virulent human culture in lieu of a BCG anti-tuberculosis vaccine, and 80 infants perished.[14] Intriguingly, although O'Donovan and the 'practicing surgeon' claimed no knowledge of the Ring incident, they readily assigned blame to the suppliers of the antigen, and instanced a recent immunization accident to back up their claim.

On 20 February, O'Farrell telephoned Saunders, conceding ignorance of the Ring incident, and relaying subsequent confirmation by college authorities that 17 children suffered adverse reactions following immunization treatment there. The college had re-opened the previous month, but seven treated children failed to return to school. O'Farrell contacted the attending physician, Daniel McCarthy, to obtain a report on the incident and forwarded a copy to Saunders. In his report, *Diphtheria immunization in Ring College*, McCarthy outlined the course of events at Ring, confirming receipt of the TAF serum from O'Farrell, the number of children treated, and the number of adverse reactions recorded.[15] However, the latter section of the report presents a detailed pathology of the affected cases, which suggests that the county pathologist, William O'Donovan, had previous knowledge of the incident. McCarthy's report ruled out 'the possibility of infection at the time of injection' and pointed to the prophylactic serum

---

13 Bonah and Menut, 'BCG vaccination, the Lübeck scandal, and the Reichsrichtlinien', in V. Roelcke and G. Maoi (eds), *Twentieth century ethics in human subjects research; historical perspectives on values, practices, and regulations* (Munchen, 2004).

14 Parish, *Victory with vaccines*, 125–26.

15 McCarthy, Report on diphtheria immunization in Ring College, 23 February 1937.

TAF as the probable cause of the reactions. In a highly scientific treatise, McCarthy suggested that Wellcome issued a serum with 'a too strong concentration of toxin [...] a too concentrated admixture of antiseptic [...] and/or a too high dosage'. McCarthy took no responsibility for the events at Ring and instead of outlining a course of treatment, his report attempted to diminish the seriousness of the incident, insisting 'all the cases are now progressing favourably, I do not anticipate any further unpleasant sequels'.[16]

On 22 February, Saunders travelled to Dungarvan to liaise with O'Farrell and McCarthy and to arrange a visit to Ring College. In a damning admission, McCarthy disclosed to Saunders that when using a syringe with a 5 c.cm barrel, he had not sterilized the syringe after use on each child, but only on each refill of serum.[17] On arrival at Ring College, it was immediately obvious to Saunders and O'Farrell that matters were not progressing as favourably as McCarthy had insisted, and both men became 'very alarmed indeed'.[18] Saunders reported that some of the children's arms were 'in a terrible state', displaying superficial granulating ulcers separated by shreds of skin in various stages of development, discharging ulcers in every case, and some degree of axillary adenitis in all. Some ulcers had been discharging since December and showed little or no healing, but peculiarly, according to McCarthy, some ulcers had developed as recently as February. Despite his unrivalled experience as an immunologist, Saunders was at a loss to explain how these cases resulted from pyrogenic injection.

On his return to Cork, Saunders received an urgent message to contact Dr Carney, physician to the Cussen family. One of the Cussen children had deteriorated, forcing Carney to perform an emergency operation to remove an enlarged axillary gland. Furthermore, Carney was now 'in no doubt that they were tubercular'. Saunders brought a sample of the child's gland to O'Donovan at UCC, and laboratory analysis confirmed beyond doubt the presence of tubercle bacilli.[19] Although he had no proof, Saunders strongly suspected that the condition that he saw in the children at Ring College, and possibly in those children unable to return to the school, was tuberculosis also. In every case, the symptoms were quite similar. Each child developed a sore arm almost at the same time, around Christmas Day.[20] In every case, an ulcer developed on the right arm, at the penetration spot of the needle. Every child developed a running sore, along with tenderness or hardness of the arm.

16 McCarthy, Report on Ring College.
17 J. C. Saunders, Letter to Richard O'Brien, Wellcome Physiological Research Laboratory, Beckenham, 23 February 1937.
18 Saunders, Letter to Richard O'Brien, 23 February 1937.
19 Saunders, Letter to Richard O'Brien, 23 February 1937.
20 WA/PP/JRH/A/75: Box 8, Robert Percy McDonnell, Notes on Dungarvan outbreak.

Serious questions remained; why were some children affected, and why did others escape injury? More importantly, if the infection was tuberculous, under what circumstances did the contaminant gain access to the serum? As Burroughs Wellcome manufactured the TAF serum used at Ring, Saunders sent a personal letter to the director of the Wellcome Physiological Research Laboratories, Richard O'Brien, to inform him of events in Waterford. Interestingly, Saunders sent the letter from his home address as he deemed the matter 'too serious to become public knowledge at the Cork public health department'. O'Brien was in America at the time; but a reply from John Trevan immediately threw suspicion on McCarthy and his methods, and the 'long latent period' that preceded disclosure of the incident.[21] Saunders cautioned that McCarthy and his advisors would claim that the serum was infected before use and he advised Trevan to send a representative to Ireland to investigate the matter further.[22]

At UCC, O'Donovan undertook further analysis of samples taken from five affected children and confirmed the presence of tuberculosis in every case. In a preliminary report, O'Donovan informed Daniel McCarthy that 'we are up against the extraordinary occurrence of inoculation of tubercle in all these cases [...] I think you must take it now that they are all tuberculous and act accordingly'.[23] O'Donovan had taken the liberty to consult with his colleague, Dr Patrick Kiely, lecturer in operative surgery at UCC and a relative of McCarthy. [24] In an attempt to aid his beleaguered cousin, Kiely suggested that McCarthy 'should seriously consider the previous contamination of the bottle contents, and accordingly the more the cases approach twenty-five, the stronger the evidence. So if there are any children absent for unknown reasons it would be very desirable to follow them up'.[25] Owing to his relationship with McCarthy, and to avoid any charge of bias, Kiely suggested that O'Donovan relate the theory of previous contamination to O'Farrell in Waterford. Fearing recrimination for supplying the immunizing materials used at Ring, and for promoting active immunization throughout Waterford, O'Farrell was keen to embrace any suggestion that detracted attention from him. O'Farrell expounded at length on the previous contamination of the

21 WA/PRL/HP/Sub/33/5. John Trevan, Letter to J. C. Saunders, 25 February 1937.
22 WA/PRL/HP/Sub/33/5. J. C. Saunders, Letter to Henry Parish, 27 February 1937.
23 WA/PRL/HP/Sub/29/10. William O'Donovan, Private Preliminary Report No. 4243. Laboratories of Pathology and Bacteriology University College Cork sent from William O'Donovan to Daniel McCarthy, 26 February 1937.
24 Patrick Gaffney, 'Book review of Kiely's, Text-book of Surgery', in *Medical Alumni Newsletter 8*, University College Cork, May 2010. In his correspondence with McCarthy, O'Donovan states that he had consulted with 'P. K.'. Patrick Kiely, Professor of Surgery at UCC was according to one of his students in Gaffney's article 'widely known as "P. K."'.
25 O'Donovan, Private Preliminary Report No. 4243.

TAF antigen, and the 'suspect phial' theory to Robert McDonnell, chief medical advisor to the DLG&PH. Although McDonnell sought to maintain distance between his department and the incident, he travelled to Ring to undertake an 'unofficial' investigation.[26]

In a previous interview with Saunders, McCarthy divulged that, contrary to good practice, he did not record the inoculation sequence at Ring. Were it recorded, it would have been possible to match the group of affected children with the exact bottle or bottles of antigen used to treat them. McCarthy's oversight frustrated retrospective efforts to establish a definite sequence, baffling the deductive skills of both Saunders and O'Farrell. However, the departmental inspector who accompanied McDonnell on his visit to Ring, John MacCormack, claimed to have succeeded where his colleagues failed; in the sense that he successfully established a definite sequence of inoculation and that 'twenty-four' affected children received serum 'from one phial of Burroughs Wellcome antigen'. Although MacCormack's investigation could not determine a definite succession among the infected cases, by attacking the problem from another angle, he surmised 'a definite succession amongst the unaffected cases' and concluded that every infected child received treatment from the same phial of antigen during the morning session on 24 November.[27] MacCormack's 'findings' so closely matched Kiely's 'suspect phial' theory that it seems more than coincidental. In his subsequent report to McDonnell, MacCormack argued 'One must suspect that first bottle used on the last day at Ring [...] it is not for us to explain how a bottle of tubercle bacillus could find its way into a bottle of TAF. There are accidents-there is sabotage'.[28]

By the end of February, the plan conceived by Kiely and O'Donovan came full circle. Reports filtered through to Saunders that a further seven children treated at Ring were reported ill,[29] and soon after, a connection was being made between the number of affected children and the number of inoculations stated on the label of a single phial of Burroughs Wellcome TAF. The suggestion that 24 children became infected after treatment with antigen extracted from one contaminated phial began to emerge in Dungarvan, and soon after, the ghost of the Lübeck disaster was evoked to support claims that the 'suspect phial' in question was mistakenly issued by Burroughs Wellcome containing a suspension of live tubercle bacilli, instead of the anti-diphtheria antigen TAF.[30]

26 McDonnell, Notes on Dungarvan.
27 *Irish Press*, 14 June 1937.
28 McDonnell, *Notes on Dungarvan*, 4.
29 WA/PRL/HP/Sub/33/5. J. C. Saunders, Letter to John Trevan, 1 March 1937.
30 Saunders, Letter to Trevan, 1 March 1937.

With the focus now shifting to Burroughs Wellcome, Saunders again contacted Trevan urging Wellcome, as a matter of urgency, to send represent-atives to investigate the matter themselves. On 6 March, Henry Parish, principal bacteriologist at the Wellcome laboratories, arrived in Cork.[31] During the fifty-mile journey from Cork to Dungarvan, Saunders updated Parish on events as they had unfolded. Over lunch in Dungarvan, Parish noted that O'Farrell remained quiet, and only spoke to express his concern regarding his own position in the event of a legal action. However, on meeting Daniel McCarthy for the first time, Parish noted 'he looked like the villain of a melodrama'.[32] McCarthy informed Parish that 24 children reported adverse reactions to Wellcome's immunizing agent, and then made the astonishing admission that, apart from the Cussen family in Cork, no other parents were aware that their children were tubercular. Parents knew that their children had 'bad arms' but they did not know how bad they were, nor did they suspect tuberculosis. The headmaster at Ring College, Séamus Ó hEocha, either through loyalty to McCarthy or fear of recrimination, probably both, concealed the severity of the children's lesions from their parents. Furthermore, Ó hEocha devised a scheme whereby students remained at Ring College to attend 'special holiday classes' over the Easter vacation, in a bid to prevent parents 'getting to know too much'.[33] Children who would have benefited from an arm sling were not accommodated, as it may have 'made the parents or locals more suspicious of serious trouble', and children who remained absent from school with lesions were in all probability attended by doctors who did not know the true nature of their patients' illness.[34]

On their return to Cork, Parish and Saunders received a visit from Patrick Kiely and William O'Donovan. Kiely admitted previous knowledge of the Ring incident, but because of 'the publicity, operative interference would entail', he conceded that 'he had not done what was in the best interest of the children'. Furthermore, he admitted that at least two children should have had lesions scraped and axillary glands removed. However, as these procedures necessitated parental consent, Kiely argued that any intervention would have been 'prejudicial to the headmaster's desire to hush things up', and did not intervene. Diverting attention from his own involvement in the cover-up, and to further exonerate his beleaguered cousin, Kiely drew attention to the 'coincidence' that 24 children succumbed to illness at Ring and that each Burroughs Wellcome phial of TAF contained 25 doses. In addition, he invoked MacCormack's sequence of inoculation among the

---

31 *British Medical Journal* (5 June 1937), 1183.
32 WA/WF/L/02/27. Confidential Report on Dr Parish's visit to Cork, March 1937.
33 Parish, Visit to Cork 1937, 2–6. See also, *Munster Express*, 17 April 1936.
34 Parish, Visit to Cork 1937, 2–6.

affected children, and concluded that all were administered TAF drawn from one phial of Burroughs Wellcome antigen.[35]

Parish rejected Kiely's assertions and MacCormack's findings on the basis that he himself, Saunders, and O'Farrell failed to establish the inoculation sequence or to substantiate the 'suspect phial' theory. Since McCarthy claimed he only prepared a nominal roll, it proved impossible to reconstruct what happened at Ring in November. Kiely then asserted that he was at a loss to explain how a dirty syringe could have given rise to 24 cases, or why McCarthy would have undertaken a scheme of inoculation which involved his own children 'in a haphazard manner'. When taking his leave, Kiely politely informed Parish 'that if there should be a case and we appeared on opposite sides, I hope that there would be no personal ill will'.[36]

On 8 March, Parish met with Robert McDonnell in Dublin. Parish invited McDonnell to inspect Wellcome laboratories to satisfy himself that the preparation of their products 'was all that could be desired', and to hold an impartial inquiry.[37] However, McDonnell, who rode in the same troop as Winston Churchill in the Sudan, and subsequently became a Colonel in both the Royal Army Medical Corp and the Irish Army Medical Corp, recognized an impending skirmish when he saw one. He determined to stay out of this one.[38] McDonnell insisted that inoculations undertaken at Ring were under a private agreement between McCarthy and the administrators of Ring College, and as they did not constitute part of a local authority immunization scheme, McDonnell declined the invitation to visit Wellcome, or to instigate an official inquiry.[39]

Furthermore, rather than broaching the previous contamination theory, McDonnell and his senior inspector Dr Winslow Sterling-Berry spoke highly of Burroughs Wellcome, and their products, and congratulated Parish on their innovative 'one-shot' APT anti-diphtheria antigen. Parish was 'suitably impressed by McDonnell's encouraging interview' and to further bolster McDonnell's support of Wellcome and their products, he offered to inject himself or his own child with any companion bottle of Burroughs Wellcome TAF which could be obtained from O'Farrell in Waterford. McDonnell assured Parish that the DLG&PH had already examined the contents of a companion bottle of TAF with negative results.

It was not in central health's best interests to have Burroughs Wellcome and their products under suspicion. McCarthy procured the antigen utilized

---

35 Parish, Visit to Cork 1937, 2–6.
36 Parish, Visit to Cork 1937, 2–6.
37 *Cork Examiner*, 15 February 1939.
38 James Deeny, *To cure and to care: Memoirs of a chief medical officer* (Dublin, 1989), 69.
39 Parish, Visit to Cork 1937, 16–19.

at Ring from local government stock, and by 1937, almost 100,000 Irish children presented for treatment to schemes using Burroughs Wellcome anti-diphtheria products. McDonnell informed Parish that he interviewed McCarthy in Dungarvan, and maintained 'some material facts of the Ring case were being concealed'.[40] McDonnell's parting comments to Parish suggested that as far his department was concerned McCarthy was on his own.

By early April, the 'hush hush' policy surrounding the Ring incident ended with fatal consequences. Despite the purchase of a violet ray lamp, most affected children showed little or no signs of healing. The Cussens threatened legal proceedings, and the condition of one child, Siobhán O'Cionnfaola, 'had become hopeless'.[41] An increasingly anxious McCarthy contacted Patrick Kiely to assist in treating the girl. When Kiely saw her on 16 April, she was 'dangerously ill', and noting the presence of bleeding patches under her skin, he called on O'Donovan to undertake bacterio-logical examinations.[42] On 19 April, Kiely and O'Donovan performed a blood transfusion on the child, but she died the next day.[43] The death of Siobhán O'Cionnfaola led to the public disclosure of the Ring incident and the impending inquest excited gossip all over Waterford, with the grave accusation that 'the best had not been done for the children'. Furthermore, the concealment of the affair did not reflect well on McCarthy, and many in Dungarvan openly blamed him for the child's death.[44]

McCarthy was born in Dungarvan, the son of a local headmaster; his family were well known and respected, and he was one of the district's leading medical practitioners. Although he tried to continue as normal, local ill will made his life 'a perpetual hell'. He received no mercy from his fellow practitioners either, some of whom took every opportunity to slander their beleaguered colleague.[45] His former medical school classmates Patrick Fitzpatrick, Cork city tuberculosis officer, and Christopher McSweeney of Cork Street Fever Hospital, Dublin, claimed McCarthy was 'the most unpopular bounder of his year' and that 'besides being a rotter, he was dirty and untidy and went about half-shaven, with dirty hands'.[46] McSweeney in particular thought that McCarthy was capable of 'any degree of sloven-liness in his work; sepsis to be expected'.[47] Regardless of the outcome of the

40 Parish, Visit to Cork 1937, 19.
41 WA/WF/L/02/27. Henry Parish, Accident at Ring, near Dungarvan, Co. Waterford, 10.
42 *Cork Examiner*, 10 February 1939.
43 *British Medical Journal* (5 June 1937), 1182.
44 Parish, Accident at Ring, 11.
45 Parish, Accident at Ring, 13.
46 WA/WF/L/02/27. Richard O'Brien, I. F. S. Ring, Confidential Report, 4.
47 O'Brien, I. F. S. Ring, Confidential Report, 4.

impending inquest, McCarthy accepted that his career in Waterford was all but finished. His wife and nine children knew nothing of the trouble hanging over him, and out of fear for their safety, they relocated to a summer bungalow outside Dungarvan.[48]

However, McCarthy had friends in high places; and mainly due to the efforts of the dogmatic Kiely, national expert opinion steadily reached consensus that Burroughs Wellcome, and not McCarthy, were at fault. Kiely, O'Donovan, and MacCormack publicly repeated the mantra that Burroughs Wellcome were culpable for the tragedy, and gained the support of the highly influential Professor W. D. O'Kelly, Department of Pathology, University College, Dublin. Although O'Kelly previously spoke highly of the Burroughs Wellcome facilities at Beckenham, which he inspected personally, both he and MacCormack engaged in 'a serious and open discussion' on the question of sabotage, asserting that 'in America and elsewhere, sacked employees did the wildest things for redress'. O'Kelly examined 30 batches of TAF antigen used at Ring, and found nothing; however, he increasingly maintained that some 'mental defective', most probably in the employ of a rival manufacturer, deliberately undertook an act of sabotage to discredit Burroughs Wellcome.

Realizing that efforts to vindicate McCarthy were gaining momentum among a group of influential physicians, Parish again lobbied Robert McDonnell to instigate an impartial inquiry, promising fullest cooperation from Wellcome. The request fell on deaf ears; again, refused on the basis that the department played no role in the Ring inoculations. Parish argued that the DLG&PH should take some responsibility because the serum used at Ring was acquired by O'Farrell, a medical officer under McDonnell's control, for a scheme approved by his department. Saunders also advised McDonnell that the matter was of national importance and that the department's failure to take charge was 'a grave mistake'. However, McDonnell remained resolute and maintained a personal and departmental distance from the Ring incident.[49]

Inquest at Ring

On 21 April 1937, Henry Parish returned to Ring to attend the inquest, which began with an autopsy on the body of Siobhán O'Cionnfaola. As Daniel McCarthy was coroner for the area, this occasion necessitated a visit by Dr T. C. Williams, coroner for Clonmel, and Dr C. J. Walsh, coroner for East Waterford. Walsh agreed in advance to postpone the inquest for a

48 Parish, Accident at Ring, 11.
49 Parish, Accident at Ring, 11.

month, so that all interested parties could collect their evidence and appoint representatives. Although the findings were not made public immediately, the post-mortem determined that acute generalized tuberculosis was the cause of death. Although McCarthy undertook the examination at the O'Cionnfaola family home, he could not bring himself to disclose the cause of death to her parents. An unidentified local doctor who reportedly 'had one or two' informed the deceased girl's father, Mícheál O'Cionnfaola, of the coroners' findings and insisted that McCarthy had been solely responsible for his daughter's death.[50] This was a great cause of concern for the grieving O'Cionnfaola family as three of their sons had also fallen ill following the inoculations at Ring College. Furthermore, in a confidential report to central health, McCarthy expressed his fears that 'systemic infection may also occur in other cases [...] and that optimism in prognosis must be tempered by grave anxiety for at least a further period of six months'.[51] Following the disclosure of the post-mortem findings, Parish wrote 'Today has been a nightmare. McCarthy is a nervous wreck and all others concerned are extremely worried. The result of the post mortem has come as a shock and a surprise and has been the last straw. A frightened and hopeless attitude is exhibited all around now'.[52]

On his return to Beckenham, Henry Parish briefed Richard O'Brien on developments in Ireland. The gravity of the position was not lost on O'Brien who was certain that when the whole story became public, legal actions for damages would be many. O'Brien was aware that a major difficulty that Wellcome faced lay in convincing Irish medical men that a fellow practitioner, even a careless one, could have infected 24 children, and Wellcome's production methods would come under suspicion.[53] With regard to the impending O'Cionnfaola inquest, O'Brien also considered the problem of convincing a jury 'who may not want to be convinced', of Burroughs Wellcome's incorruptibility. In light of this, he decided that an Irish jury should hear Wellcome's evidence from Irish voices.

O'Brien requested W. J. Bigger, Professor of Bacteriology, Trinity College, Dublin, to carry out a detailed inspection of operations at Wellcome's Beckenham facility and to appear as a witness at the inquest of Siobhan O'Cionnfaola. When O'Brien intimated that Wellcome might not have representation at the inquest, Bigger advised that 'Irish juries have a habit, in actions involving English and others, of being extraordinarily sympathetic

50 Parish, Accident at Ring, 11.
51 WF/M/GB/01/37/01. Daniel McCarthy, Private and Confidential Report from Dr McCarthy to Department of Local Government and Public Health on complications following TAF inoculations at Ring College Co. Waterford.
52 Parish, Accident at Ring, 12.
53 WA/WF/L/02/27. Richard O'Brien, General Notes.

with the poor little Irishman fighting a rich English or foreign firm and of giving curious verdicts in favour of the local men, irrespective of the evidence'.[54] Bigger advised that it might be prudent to convey to the coroner the suggestion that the best verdict would be 'death from purpura caused by tubercle arising from injection'. Bigger's suggestion alarmed O'Brien. He was convinced that McCarthy and the college headmaster, Ó hEocha, would suppress any mention of tuberculosis at the inquest. Bigger asserted that too many people knew the whole affair and that there was a very real possibility that more affected children would die. He further suggested that a jury might bring in a ruling that the child's death was due to the injection of a prophylactic issued in a contaminated form from Burroughs Wellcome, and in such a ruling, there would be no chance of an appeal. O'Brien took Bigger's comments seriously, acted accordingly, and took steps to ensure that both legal and medical representatives would attend the inquest on Wellcome's behalf.[55]

On 18 May 1937, the inquest into the death of Siobhán O'Cionnfaola resumed at the Vocational School, Ring, with Dr C. J. Walsh, coroner for East Waterford residing.[56] From the outset, Walsh expressed his concern that he was conducting the inquest out of jurisdiction. McCarthy was the coroner for West Waterford; however, his role as a necessary witness at the inquest debarred him from acting in that capacity. McCarthy's deputy, T. C. Williams was a legal advisor to McCarthy and thereby debarred from acting as coroner also. Walsh assumed that his jurisdiction was therefore in order and swore in a jury of nine local men with William Meehan as foreman. Since Ring is located in a Gaeltacht area of Ireland, it was necessary to translate proceedings through Irish for the benefit of jurors, and for Mícheál O'Cionnfaola, who had not spoken English for twenty years previously. Walsh informed those present that he first opened the inquest on 21 April, the day after the child's death, and on that occasion, he had merely taken formal evidence of identification from Mícheál O'Cionnfaola, and a statement from William O'Donovan in his capacity as county pathologist.[57]

On swearing in, O'Donovan revealed the full results of the post-mortem examination. He stated that 'certain organs' revealed traces of tubercle bacilli

54 WA/WF/L/02/27. Richard O'Brien, I. F. S. Professor Bigger, 17 May 1937.
55 O'Brien, I. F. S. Professor Bigger, 17 May 1937.
56 *Dungarvan Observer*, 22 May 1937. Legal representation: T. J. Kelly, State Solicitor, Wexford, and Supt. M. Walsh conducted proceedings for the State. Mr. D. Fawcett, appeared for Ring College authorities. Mr T. C. Williams appeared for Daniel McCarthy; Mr E. A. Ryan for Mícheál O' Cionnfaola, J. J. Sheehy, and J. Desmond; Mr J. J. Horgan for Burroughs Wellcome; and Mr James Mooney for an 'interested party'.
57 *Dungarvan Observer*, 22 May 1937.

in the lung, liver, spleen, kidney, and glands, and although the appearance of the ulcerated lesion on the right arm was consistent with a tuberculous ulcer, no trace of tubercular bacilli was found there.[58] He further stated that there was no evidence of chronic tuberculosis, and that the cause of the disease was a tuberculous ulcer, disseminated throughout the body, leading to purpuric haemorrhage, 'possibly as a result of the introduction of a living tuberculosis serum'.[59] Under cross-examination, O'Donovan conceded that there was a possible connection between the death of Siobhán O'Cionnfaola from general miliary tuberculosis, and the inoculation into the right arm some months previously.[60]

An investigation into the method of sterilization implemented at Dungarvan district hospital, where McCarthy procured the syringes used at Ring College, focused on the theatre sister, Sister Oliver, who followed routine procedure there. She disassembled the syringes used by McCarthy, boiled them for an hour in an electric sterilizer, lifted them with sterilized forceps and immersed them in absolute alcohol until needed. When required for use, she wrapped the syringes in a sterile swab, and put them in a sterile towel for conveyance.[61] The attending nurse at Ring College, Elizabeth Denn, stated that McCarthy used the same three syringes in both the Friary school and Ring College and employed the same immunization technique in both locations.[62] She described how McCarthy assembled a syringe with needle, washed it in ether and alcohol, touched the rubber seal on the phials of TAF with the disinfectant Lysol, washed the arm of each child with ether and applied alcohol to the site of penetration. Contrary to McCarthy's admission to Saunders in Dungarvan, Denn stated that McCarthy dipped the syringe needle in alcohol between each injection, and kept iodine ready in case of bleeding.[63] The fact that no streptococcal or other infection occurred suggests that the method of sterilization utilized at Dungarvan district hospital, and the technique employed by McCarthy, had indeed been sound.

The question of culpability then shifted to the Wellcome laboratories and the materials utilized in the Ring inoculations. Richard O'Brien stated that Wellcome issued 320 25 c.cm bottles of batch P.521 anti-diphtheria serum TAF on 11 November 1935. This batch treated over 7,000 children throughout Britain and Ireland, with no other reactions reported. The supposition that a single phial became infected and was responsible for causing 24 adverse reactions was a serious charge; however, O'Brien argued

58 'A fatality after diphtheria immunization', *British Medical Journal* (5 June 1937), 1182.
59 *British Medical Journal* (5 June 1937), 1183.
60 *Dungarvan Observer*, 22 May 1937, 1.
61 *Cork Examiner*, 8 February 1939.
62 McDonnell, Notes on Dungarvan, 2.
63 *Dungarvan Observer*, 22 May 1937, 5.

that 'while that hypothesis needed to be examined', a second hypothesis which required close examination was the possibility that the serum become infected locally at Ring.[64] O'Brien outlined how he and Henry Parish traced every bottle of TAF from batch P.521, tracking progress through every stage of production, which as good practice dictated, was recorded on cards. They found no possibility of contamination of a bottle of TAF with living tubercle bacilli. Furthermore, O'Brien asserted that even if such an accident occurred, research undertaken by Douglas and Hartley decisively proved that living tubercle could not survive for more than 48 hours in a suspension comprised of 0.5 per cent phenol.[65] Professor O'Kelly confirmed that 20 phials of batch P.521 from Michael O'Farrell's local government stock contained the recommended amount of phenol, and contemporary medical opinion agreed it would have been impossible for tubercle bacillus to survive in such a mixture. Further tests at Wellcome laboratories intentionally introduced living tubercle bacilli into a sample batch of P.521 antigen. A culture derived immediately from the material gave profuse growth of bacilli, those made after 24 hours yielded very little, and those cultures made after seven days produced none. When injected with the mixture, no laboratory animal developed tuberculosis. Wellcome repeated the same experiments with a culture obtained from one of the affected children and obtained the same results; the living tubercle bacilli introduced into batch P.521, died in less than 48 hours.[66]

Speculation then shifted to the possibility that Wellcome supplied a bottle of tubercle bacillus with a TAF label mistakenly affixed. Adopting this line of inquiry, Mr Ryan, solicitor for Micheál O'Cionnfaola, asked Professor Bigger if there were any suspicions that the TAF serum used to immunize children at Ring College could have been 'criminally interfered with'.[67] Bigger acknowledged that he considered the possibility of 'deliberate sabotage', and communicated his concerns to Richard O'Brien. However, they concluded that it would have been 'impossible for a stranger to infiltrate the laboratories to do the criminal act'.[68] Continuing with his cross-examination, Ryan asserted that in England, acts of sabotage were 'not committed by strangers but by inside employees, usually in the employ of rival manufacturers wishing to bring their competitors into disrepute'. While

64 WF/M/GB/01/37/1. Richard O'Brien, Notes on accident at Ring, 4 May 1937.
65 Douglas, S. R. and Percival Hartley, 'The preparation of old tuberculin by the use of synthetic media with observations on its properties and stability'. *Tubercle*, Vol. 16 (1935), 105–13.
66 O'Brien, Notes on Ring.
67 'Remarkable evidence; Possibility of interference with serum', *Irish Independent*, 22 May 1937.
68 *Dungarvan Observer*, 29 May 1937.

Bigger acknowledged that such incidents had not been unknown, he stressed that in this case it was unlikely that any rival firm would benefit, because the product in question was mainly used for children and 'if one firm is hit, all are hit'.[69]

Under further questioning, Bigger gave evidence that he inspected the research laboratories at the Wellcome Foundation Ltd, Kent. He insisted that he was afforded 'every facility for investigation' at the laboratories, where he followed the various stages in the preparation of TAF and inspected records dealing with the batches of antigen from which the flasks used at Ring originated. Bigger assured the jury that TAF manufactured at Wellcome was 'at every point free from contamination, as it was tested microscopically, culturally, and by animal inoculation'. He was satisfied from his inspection 'that no tubercle bacilli could have been added to a bottle of TAF'. In relation to the charge that a possible substitution of a bottle of tubercle bacilli for a bottle of TAF had occurred, Bigger stated that he found 'no sufficient motive to impel anyone to make such a substitution', and that any attempt to do so at Wellcome laboratories 'would have been faced with insurmountable difficulty'.[70]

Mr J. J. Horgan, representing Burroughs Wellcome, explained to the jury that when Wellcome manufactured TAF, it was stored in four-litre bottles. Horgan reasoned that if something contaminated the serum during the production stages, that this would have affected hundreds of bottles, and not just one. Regarding the charge of 'malicious substitution', Horgan stated that he could not understand why 'a madman or blackguard' would go to the trouble of substituting or infecting one bottle when they could not determine where that bottle would end up or 'what motive anybody could have to do such a thing'. Horgan insisted that his clients 'supplied a properly prepared article and their connection with the case ceased there'. He further asserted that Burroughs Wellcome's product was 'well established, proved successful', and that it would be 'a cruel tragedy if the lives of future children were sacrificed through any public panic at the use of this material'.[71]

When called as a witness, Henry Parish produced records relating to batches of the P.521 antigen used at Ring College, demonstrating that they had passed all tests on repeated occasions.[72] Parish pointed out that during the period in which McCarthy undertook the Ring College immunizations Michael O'Farrell had used 30 bottles of antigen from the same batch of antigen in Waterford without any ill effects. In addition, Parish produced

69   *Irish Independent*, 22 May 1937.
70   *Irish Independent*, 22 May 1937.
71   *Irish Press*, 14 June 1937.
72   *British Medical Journal* (5 June 1937), 1182.

the results of three separate bacteriological examinations undertaken by Wellcome laboratories, Dr O'Donovan of University College, Cork, and Dr O'Kelly of the National University on samples of leftover antigen supplied by Dr McCarthy, and on the remaining supplies of TAF held by O'Farrell. In every case, specimens of antigen examined at all three laboratories produced a negative result, and none found any trace of tubercule bacilli.[73]

Addressing the possibility that a single bottle of P.521 antigen became infected at Ring prior to use, Horgan argued that material from a patient with active tuberculosis could contaminate the barrel of a syringe, or a towel on which the barrel was placed after sterilization, and spoke of two cases where such occurrences had previously been proved. In one instance, a case involving the intravenous injection of Salvarsan as a remedy for syphilis resulted in fatalities as the first man treated had malaria. This man's contaminated blood adhered to the tubing of the syringe, the ten succeeding men became infected, and some fatalities ensued.[74]

In the second incident, a group of nurses who received anti-diphtheria treatment each developed an abscess at the site of inoculation, and many were gravely ill for some days. Bacterial examination identified the presence of streptococci in every case and doctors traced the source of infection to the throat of the nurse who had handled the syringes. Samples of the streptococci died within a few days when introduced into a sample of the prophylactic, proving that the contaminant had not been in the serum when issued. The offending nurse accidentally infected the saline solution in which the syringes lay ready for use, subsequently causing the infection of many nurses. Horgan asserted that pathologists might find these events to be 'surprising if not incredible' but the evidence strongly suggested that the contamination of TAF used at Ring could well have occurred in a similar way, particularly in the presence of heavy local infection.[75]

During the inquest, an article appeared in the *Daily Mirror* stating that serum used at Ring College had been manufactured in the 'Free State laboratories' and that this opinion was 'widely held in Waterford and neighbouring counties'.[76] The article further asserted that the affected children received inoculation treatment six months previously with the serum prepared 'in an Irish laboratory'. The author of the piece based his assertions on an interview he conducted with Professor Bigger, who it was claimed, stated that the error that caused the death of Siobhán O'Cionnfaola and the illness of the

73 McDonnell, Notes on Dungarvan outbreak, 1.
74 J. B. Black, 'The accidental transmission of malaria through intravenous injections of op neoarsphenamine', *American Journal of Epidemiology*, Vol. 31 Section C, No. 2 (1940), 37–42.
75 O'Brien, Notes on Ring.
76 *Irish Independent*, 12 June 1937.

other children 'was not made in the laboratory of Burroughs Wellcome'. In addition, the *Daily Mirror* stated that 24 children were affected, that they had been examined and proved to be suffering from tuberculosis, and that all patients were believed to be 'seriously ill, and incurable'.[77]

In a voluntary statement, Bigger admitted that he had partaken in a telephone interview with the London representative of the *Daily Mirror*, who informed him that the report of the inquest they received had been 'short and scrappy'. Mr D. Fawcett, representing the authorities of Ring College, forcefully argued that the newspaper report, and Bigger's input in particular, was an act of contempt of the coroners' court. Fawcett asserted that the publication of such an article was 'a travesty' insomuch as it 'misrepresented all material facts except the death of one child', and that it caused a great deal of pain and anxiety to the parents of children who fell ill because of the inoculation they received. Bigger apologized to the coroner and the jury, and denied any intention of infringing on their rights. Dr Walsh agreed that the article was not only 'outrageous' but also 'grossly inaccurate' and that the only explanation for its appearance was that it was 'a deliberately malicious report'.[78]

Summing up, Mr Fawcett stated that his client Dr McCarthy impressed counsel 'as a man, sincere and honest, who had not hidden anything', who used serum supplied to him which bore the name Burroughs Wellcome, London, 'a firm of the highest repute as manufacturing chemists', without investigating its content. Fawcett asserted that immunization was adopted 'practically universally [...] had been counselled and advised by medical authorities [...] and it was therefore the duty of those entrusted with the care of children at Ring College to take every precaution to safeguard the health of the children entrusted to them'. Fawcett cautioned the jury that they had a duty to bring in something more than an open verdict, stressing that they had a duty to bring in a verdict 'placing the responsibility for the death of this child on the proper shoulders'.[79]

As far as J. J. Horgan, was concerned, nothing had come out which would make an action for damages. He thought the case had gone well and he did not see how Burroughs Wellcome could have an adverse decision against them. However, Horgan did ask the jury to confine their verdict to the cause of death 'as only an expert tribunal could properly judge the other issues'.[80] When evidence concluded, the coroner Dr Walsh reviewed

77 *Dungarvan Observer*, 19 June 1937.
78 *Irish Independent*, 12 June 1937.
79 *Irish Press*, 14 June 1937.
80 WF/L/02/09. J. J. Horgan, Letter to Markby, Stewart, and Wadesons, Solicitors, 14 June 1937.

the circumstances leading up to the inquest and put the following questions to the jury:

> When, where, and why did the deceased die?
> Was the ulcer on her arm a tuberculous ulcer?
> If it was a tuberculous ulcer, did the general tuberculous condition from which she died spread from this?
> If it was a tuberculous ulcer, did the microbes causing it enter the body at the time the child was inoculated against diphtheria? If they did enter it at the time, what was their source and how did they come to be injected? [81]

At several intervals during the inquest, Walsh raised the question of his jurisdiction on the basis that he was neither coroner nor deputy coroner for the Dungarvan area, and at this point, he decided to send the depositions to the Department of Justice in Dublin and to await their directions, before resuming to give a verdict. The Minister for Justice, P. J. Ruttledge, directed to appoint Dr Walsh as deputy coroner for West Waterford in a temporary capacity, thereby regularizing his eligibility to oversee the final inquest proceedings.[82] Walsh had become uneasy as the hearing progressed. Whether the highly scientific nature of the arguments presented made him feel out of his depth or whether he became cognisant of an impending controversial verdict, Walsh made every attempt to shirk his responsibility as coroner. He intimated that the jury could only answer questions put to them definitively through a 'long, searching, and highly scientific investigation', better suited 'to a body of scientists rather than a coroner's jury'.[83] Addressing the jury Walsh stated: 'If you believe gentlemen that you are not in a position to give an opinion as to the origin of the tubercle bacilli, you will say so, and I cannot see how you are in such a position'.[84] After a short deliberation, a verdict brought by the jury concluded:

> We, the members of the Coroner's jury, unanimously agree with the medical testimony that Siobhán Kennealy [O'Cionnfaola] died on April 20th, 1937, from toxaemia [sic] and purpuric haemorrhage, consequent to general miliary tuberculosis infection, and that we are of opinion according to the evidence placed before us that the tuberculous condition was originated by the inoculation of prophylactic into the

---

81 *Dungarvan Observer*, 19 June 1937, 3.
82 *Dungarvan Observer*, 19 June 1937, 3.
83 'Protracted inquest concludes at Ring', *Munster Express*, 18 June 1937.
84 *Munster Express*, 18 June 1937.

right arm of Siobhan Kennealy in Nov., 1936, and that we are of the opinion that the contents of the 25c.c. bottle of prophylactic labelled TAF Burroughs and Wellcome, from which a portion of the material was extracted by Dr Daniel McCarthy, for the purpose of the aforesaid inoculation, contained tubercle bacilli, and that the inoculation was carried out by Dr McCarthy according to the most approved surgical technique. Every precaution was taken by him to guard against infection arising from contaminated surgical appliances, and we exonerate him from all blame in this matter.[85]

Walsh clearly underestimated the mental capacity of the 'not very well educated country people' of the jury. Although comprised of Irish speaking farmers, fishermen, local tradesmen, and shopkeepers,[86] they demonstrated a thorough comprehension of the lengthy and complex medico-legal arguments placed before them and brought in a comprehensive verdict. Or, it may have been the fact that all nine jurors, as J. J. Horgan argued, 'had demonstrated an intense desire to whitewash McCarthy and to prevent injury to Ring College'.[87]

In a small and close-knit community, such as Ring, the college had crucial implications for the local economy. Such a large facility, housing 100 boarding students and teaching staff, was not only an important local employer, but it was the greatest consumer of local goods and services in the area. It was no surprise that a jury comprised of local men whose livelihoods relied on the continued patronage of Ring College would embrace any conclusion that averted a negative economic impact.[88] With regard to McCarthy, he was after all 'one of their own'. He and his family were well known and respected in West Waterford. He was a family man with a wife and children to support,[89] and it seems reasonable to assume that the jury was comprised of either friends or patrons of 'Doctor Dan'. If we further consider that, the foreman of the jury, William Meehan, was a brother in-law of Séamus Ó hEocha, the college principal, it becomes clear that the difficulty of getting an impartial inquiry at Ring had been fraught with insurmountable difficulties.[90] The multinational organization was no match for Irish small-town politics, and

---

85 *Dungarvan Observer*, 19 June 1937.
86 J. J. Horgan, Letter to Markby, Stewart, and Wadesons, Solicitors, 14 June 1937.
87 Horgan, Letter to Markby, Stewart, and Wadesons, Solicitors, 14 June 1937.
88 Olwen Purdue, 'The Irish Poor Law in a north Antrim town, 1861–1921', *Irish Historical Studies*, Vol. XXXVII, No. 148 (November 2011), 567–83.
89 WF/M/GB/01/37/01. J. J. Horgan, Interview with Nurse Elizabeth Denn, 8 October 1938.
90 WF/L/02/09, J. J. Horgan, Letter to Markby, Stewart, and Wadesons, Solicitors, 1 July 1937.

Horgan was convinced that the laws of evidence and the legal position 'had been undermined by local prejudice'. In a personal correspondence to Henry Parish, Horgan, in less than charming language, demonstrated his frustration by exclaiming, 'I am convinced that the nigger [*sic*] in the woodpile was at Ring and that whatever took place, took place there, but I do not believe that anything will ever be proved'.[91] Horgan was of the opinion that as a teacher at Ring College, Micheál O'Cionnfaola 'would not have the means to embark on an expensive and speculative litigation'. O'Cionnfaola himself had to weigh up his desire for justice and recompense for the loss of his daughter, against his desire to protect Ring College, an institution he co-founded, and the means through which he supported his wife and nine children. The inquest findings absolved the college authorities of any blame, and any further action ran the risk of attracting further bad publicity, which would do little to repair the already damaged reputation of the college. It seems likely that the college principal Séamus Ó hEocha was happy to let the matter lie. However, on 9 August, Micheál O' Cionnfaola initiated high court proceedings against Dr Daniel McCarthy, and the Wellcome Foundation Ltd, 'for loss sustained by him by reason of the death of his daughter Siobhán O' Cionnfaola'.[92]

Preparing for Battle

At least three other families whose children became ill after the Ring inoculation, and who were not 'going on well' as statements by Séamus Ó hEocha suggested, employed legal representatives to attend Siobhán O'Cionnfaola's inquest. Mr E. A. Ryan, Dungarvan, represented Micheál O'Cionnfaola; however, he also represented J. J. Sheehy of Courtmacsherrry on behalf of his children, Máire and Maurice, and J. Desmond of Ballymacarbry, on behalf of his son Michael. Mr James Mooney of Babington, Clarke, and Mooney Solicitors, Cork, appeared on behalf of 'an interested party' who it may be reasonable to assume were the Cussen family on behalf of their children, Gerald and Finola.[93]

In a chance meeting between the Cussens and Jack Saunders, Mr Cussen revealed that his son Gerald, who recovered somewhat after the removal of his axillary gland some months earlier, subsequently developed 'open enlarged

---

91 WF/L/02/09. J. J. Horgan, Letter to Markby, Stewart, and Wadesons, Solicitors, 14 June 1937.
92 1937- No. 488 P. High Court of Justice.
93 WF/L/02/14. List of children immunised against diphtheria in November 1936. See also, *Dungarvan Observer*, 22 May 1936.

glands above and below the clavicle'. Cussen further claimed that several more children were 'in a serious condition', and that parents were fearful that 'there will be several further deaths to be recorded'. In correspondence with Henry Parish, Saunders informed him that parents of children affected at Ring had 'formed a union' and from what he could gather, Saunders cautioned that 'the situation was a very serious one indeed'.[94]

In response to Micheál O'Cionnfaola's legal action, parents of some affected children held a meeting in Cork to decide on what further action, if any, they should take. A report in the *Cork Examiner* stated that those present had contacted all parents of children who received immunization treatment at Ring College and their enquiries attracted 17 replies. Some parents stated that their only interest in the case was to 'expose McCarthy if possible'; as some children's analogous accounts of the proceedings suggested that, 'there had been a great degree of carelessness during the inoculations'[95]

The following week parents held a second meeting in Dungarvan. Eleven families were in attendance and a further four families forwarded letters regretting their inability to attend. Parents who attended the meeting reported that their children were doing quite well following specialist treatment. However, they all expressed general disappointment and dissatisfaction with the DLG&PH who some parents, with some justification, claimed 'had failed to show any evidence of interest in this matter of vital importance, for the families concerned, and for the children of the country as a whole'.

Many parents strongly expressed the opinion that the DLG&PH had recommended anti-diphtheria immunization to all local authorities, and it seemed 'only reasonable to expect that the department should intervene with all the resources at its disposal to assist parents in determining responsibility for the terrible calamity that had befallen their children'. As this had not transpired, the informal parents' union decided to take steps to bring the whole affair to the notice of the Minister and his department, and to have the full facts of the case submitted to all Dáil Éireann deputies.[96]

In September, a parent's deputation travelled to the Customs House, Dublin, to meet with Minister for Local Government and Public Health, Seán T. O'Kelly, to ask him to direct an inquiry into the Ring College incident.[97] Minister O'Kelly informed the delegation that the incident was 'a matter of great concern' to him and he expressed his 'greatest sympathy for the parents of the deceased child, and the parents whose children had been

94 WF/L/02/09. J. C. Saunders, Letter to Henry Parish, 24 September 1937.
95 WF/L/02/09. Letter from J. J. Horgan to Parish, 18 June 1937, letter from J. C. Saunders to Parish, 24 September 1937, and letter from J. J. Horgan to Markby, Stewart, and Wadeson, 1 November 1937.
96 *Munster Express*, 27 August 1937.
97 *Irish Independent*, 12 June 1937.

subjected to such unnecessary suffering'. O'Kelly pledged the full support of his Department to ensure that 'everything possible would be done to hasten the recovery of those children who were still affected', and stated that he was fully prepared to consider 'any proposals for affording specialised treatment for children submitted to him through local authorities'. However, O'Kelly reiterated the response previously issued to Henry Parish; the inoculation of children at Ring did not form part of an official scheme of immunization against diphtheria approved by the DLG&PH; the inoculations 'were carried out under a private arrangement with the authorities of the college', and that neither he, nor his Department, could 'intervene in regard to the treatment of private patients by a medical practitioner'.[98]

In October, a number of deputies raised questions regarding the Ring College incident in Dáil Éireann. Seamus Burke (Fine Gael) asked Minister O'Kelly if he had received a memorial from the children affected at Ring, and if his department was prepared to 'undertake an official inquiry to determine the responsibility for the occurrence, and to provide, if necessary, adequate compensation for the parents concerned'. Richard Anthony (Independent Labour) stated that the DLG&PH 'should actively interest itself in investigating the cause of the disaster that befell so many children as a result of treatment given them in accordance with the policy of the Department'.[99] W. T. Cosgrave (Fine Gael) asked the Minister whether special precautions had been taken since the circumstances surrounding Ring came to light 'to direct attention to the dangers associated with such operations, and to secure proper precautions being taken against a repetition of the occurrence'.[100] O'Kelly's response to the deputies' questions altered little from what had by then become the standard Departmental response, and a commitment to hold an official inquiry was not forthcoming.

In Cork, J. J. Horgan became aware of the parent's union and their visit to the Customs House, but the most interesting aspect to him was that just seventeen children had representation. It struck him that Daniel McCarthy never supplied proof that 24 children had experienced adverse reactions at Ring.[101] Henry Parish examined 12 children,[102] Jack Saunders identified 17,[103] O'Donovan's evidence related to 15 cases altogether,[104] and Patrick Kiely subsequently admitted that although it could not be proved that 24 children contracted tuberculosis he insisted that it was 'morally certain that they

98 Dáil Éireann, *Parliamentary Debates*, Vol. 69, 6 October 1937, 39.
99 *Parliamentary Debates*, Vol. 69, 6 October 1937, 37.
100 *Parliamentary Debates*, Vol. 69, 6 October 1937, 38.
101 WF/L/02/09, J. J. Horgan, Letter to Henry Parish, 26 June 1937.
102 WF/L/02/09, Henry Parish, Letter to J. J. Horgan, 28 June 1937.
103 Horgan to Parish, 26 June 1937.
104 WF/L/02/09, J. J. Horgan, Letter to Henry Parish, 9 July 1937.

had'.[105] When Horgan subsequently contacted Ring College to ascertain a list of children who suffered no ill effects after inoculation, the school produced a list containing 13 names: suggesting no deviation from the original assertion that 24 of 37 treated children had fallen ill. [106]

At a meeting of the British Medical Association in Belfast, a Dr Trimble reportedly told Wellcome's Dublin representative, Mr Webb, that while attending a medical conference in Bristol a doctor stated that 'he knew for a fact that McCarthy drew a cold abscess the day prior to giving the fatal injection' at Ring College.[107] Following up on Webb's report, Horgan contacted Dr Trimble in Belfast who identified the Bristol doctor as one Dr Munro. When questioned on the remark, Munro distanced himself from the assertion and transformed his remark into the definite statement that 'McCarthy had used a dirty syringe'.[108] Horgan knew that this kind of information was useless unless verified, and although he took steps to obtain more information on these points, progress proved difficult. Horgan lamented, 'everyone knows but no one will help'.[109]

In December 1938, Horgan contacted Robert McDonnell of the DLG&PH requesting copies of reports on Ring made by the departmental inspector MacCormack, and by Daniel McCarthy.[110] McDonnell's responded stating that there were no 'official reports' made by his department, and that no report on the Ring incident was forwarded by McCarthy.[111] When Horgan then asked McDonnell if any 'unofficial reports' were submitted, McDonnell stated that no correspondence was received from McCarthy regarding Ring college, and that notes made by MacCormack and McDonnell were undertaken in a 'purely personal capacity [...] and solely out of interest in the medical aspects of the case'.[112]

In an interview with Horgan, Dr Carney, physician to the Cussen children, stated that members of the parents' union were sure that Burroughs Wellcome was not responsible for what befell their children. However, they were equally convinced that the inquest verdict 'had been concocted by McCarthy's legal team and medical advisors'.[113] In a subsequent interview

105 WF/L/02/09, J. J. Horgan to Henry Parish, 9 August 1937.
106 WF/L/02/14, Michael O' Donnell, Letter to J. J. Horgan, 28 January 1939.
107 Horgan to Parish, 9 August 1937.
108 WF/L/02/09, J. J. Horgan, Letter to Markby, Stewart, and Wadesons, 13 November 1937.
109 Horgan to Parish, 9 August 1937.
110 WF/L/02/14, J. J. Horgan, Letter to R. P. McDonnell, Department of Local Government and Public Health, 2 December 1938.
111 WF/L/02/14, R. P. McDonnell, DLG&PH, Letter to J. J. Horgan, 9 December 1938.
112 WF/L/02/14, R. P. McDonnell, DLG&PH, Letter to J. J. Horgan, 17 December 1938.
113 WF/L/02/09, J. J. Horgan, Letter to Markby, Stewart, and Wadesons, 1 November 1937.

with Dr Walsh, the coroner who oversaw the inquest, Walsh revealed in confidence that he was also 'quite satisfied that the verdict was concocted outside' and expressed his annoyance that his name should be in any way connected with such a document. Furthermore, Walsh revealed that McCarthy's advisors made every effort to get him to 'adjourn the inquest indefinitely so that the matter would never be investigated'.[114]

In the weeks leading up to the High Court case, it emerged that the secretary at Ring College, Michael O'Donnell, unearthed a previously unknown list of children inoculated by McCarthy at Ring. Curiously, no mention of O'Donnell or any such list had surfaced at the inquest. When Horgan requested a copy of the list, O'Donnell informed him, that as well as the 37 children treated with TAF there were also 'a few children under seven years of age who were inoculated with a milder serum'.[115] In subsequent correspondence, O'Donnell confirmed that the younger children, Aengus Hough and Millicent McCarthy, were administered Wellcome's experimental APT vaccine.[116]

In an interview with Elizabeth Denn, the attending nurse at Ring College, Denn stated that one of the two younger children, who should have received treatment with APT, was Cullen from Wexford. However, nurse Denn stated that McCarthy mistakenly administered TAF, instead of APT, to the Cullen child and had no choice but to subsequently administer the full three doses of TAF to the child.[117] Interestingly, the children identified by O'Donnell as having received treatment with an alternative antigen were the children of the headmaster Ó hEocha (Hough), and the attending physician McCarthy.

Although the Cullen child experienced no adverse reaction following inoculation, Denn's admission revealed that McCarthy failed to disclose this element of neglect. Denn's second disclosure, which O'Donnell, the college secretary confirmed, was that McCarthy also failed to disclose that he had used a serum other than Wellcome's batch P. 521 at Ring. McCarthy and his advisors failed to disclose that 17 children, and not 24, experienced adverse reactions following treatment. McCarthy wilfully suppressed knowledge that Michael O'Donnell had witnessed the inoculations, and had taken a list of the succession in which children were treated. Department Secretary, Robert McDonnell, refuted McCarthy's claim that he had submitted a full report of the Ring incident to central health early in 1937. A most damning indictment of McCarthy, and his advisors, was the deep sense of shame expressed by the coroner, Dr Walsh, who confirmed attempted criminal interference sought

114 Horgan to Markby, Stewart, and Wadesons, 1 November 1937.
115 WF/L/02/14, Michael O' Donnell, Letter to J. J. Horgan, 19 January 1939.
116 WF/L/02/14, Michael O' Donnell, Letter to J. J. Horgan, 21 January 1939.
117 J. J. Horgan, Note of interview with Nurse Elizabeth Denn, 8 October 1938.

to obstruct the course of the inquest, and when that intervention failed, an unduly influenced, and a now implicated jury, returned a 'concocted' verdict.

However, the most disturbing evidence suggesting that a criminal conspiracy surrounded Siobhán O'Cionnfaola's death is on her gravestone in St Nicholas Chapel, at Ring. Throughout the inquest, the medical trinity of McCarthy, Kiely, and O'Donovan insisted that the child fell dangerously ill on 16 April 1936 and despite their greatest efforts, including the adminis-tration of two blood transfusions, she died four days later on 20 April 1936. However, Siobhán O'Cionnfaola's headstone states that she died on 16 April 1936, three days before the eminent physicians claim to have treated her. No other physician attended Siobhán during her illness and the results of O'Donovan's post-mortem examination went uncontested. Siobhán O'Cionnfaola became ill due to the actions of a negligent physician, and died because of his efforts to cloak that negligence. The final and most sinister move was the appropriation of her corpse in an ultimately successful attempt to vindicate those responsible for her death.

Despite a formal request to the Births, Deaths, and Marriages, and an assurance from staff at that office that they undertook two comprehensive searches, no death certificate for Siobhán O'Cionnfaola or Siobhán Kennealy was located. As far as that office is concerned, Siobhán O'Cionnfaola's death was never registered. Similarly, a perusal of coroner records at the National Archives of Ireland, and requests to the coroner's office for East and West Waterford, have failed to identify a copy of the coroner's report relating to Siobhán O'Cionnfaola's inquest.

6

O'Cionnfaola v. the Wellcome Foundation
and Daniel McCarthy

On 6 February 1939, an action taken by Micheál and Bríd O'Cionnfaola against Daniel McCarthy and the Wellcome Foundation Ltd began before the President of the High Court, Mr Justice Conor Maguire.[1] The O'Cionnfaola's claimed damages in respect of the death of their daughter, Siobhán, and in respect of loss and personal injuries sustained by their three sons, due to illness incurred following immunization treatment at Ring College. The plaintiffs alleged that the TAF preparation used during the inoculations at Ring 'was negligently prepared, manufactured, tested, or stored by the Wellcome Foundation' and issued by them to Dr Michael O'Farrell, 'containing tubercle bacilli'. The claim against Daniel McCarthy did not infer that he performed his duties in a perfunctory manner, but that he 'warranted the quality and fitness of the preparation used'.[2] Opening for the plaintiffs, E. J. Kelly stated that the case was of 'vast and critical importance'.[3] Kelly continued:

> This case is unique. It is a case whose importance touches every hospital, every medical practitioner, and every manufacturer of medical preparations. It is unique because as far as we know, no such case has ever reached the courts. It is no exaggeration to say that the reports of this case and the results of it will be greatly canvassed wherever doctors meet in the English-speaking world and, indeed, all over the world.[4]

In Britain, contemporary medical practitioners regarded the charge levelled against the Wellcome Foundation as somewhat audacious, bordering on the

---

1 'Chemist sued for child's death', *Irish Times*, 7 February 1939.
2 *Irish Times*, 7 February 1939.
3 'Drug used to inoculate children', *Cork Examiner*, 7 February 1939.
4 *Cork Examiner*, 7 February 1939.

impudent. One contributor to the *British Medical Journal* referred to the whole case as 'extraordinary', and given the reputation of the manufacturers, the charge that a preparation of TAF was contaminated when it left the laboratory, 'seems incredible'.[5] In the House of Commons, William Leach, Labour MP for Bradford, raised concern regarding the safety of Wellcome's prophylactic, asking if it was 'the same as that freely used in this country'.[6] While health minister Walter Elliott allayed parliamentarian's concerns, he instructed his department to open up a line of correspondence between Whitehall and the Custom House in Dublin. Dr J. R. Hutchinson, Deputy Senior Medical Officer at the Ministry of Health, requested a transcript of evidence presented at the High Court proceedings from his Irish counterpart Robert McDonnell, stating 'Questions in the House of Commons have already arisen out of this incident and it seems likely that we may have others. We are therefore anxious to be forearmed with as much information as we can obtain'.[7] The DLG&PH refused the request on the basis that it would cost £20 to procure. The reply must have seemed somewhat strange to Hutchinson, but it is certain that McDonnell's response further ensured that no official connection was made between his department and the Ring College incident.

On the first day of the High Court hearing, E. J. Kelly reiterated the plaintiffs' conviction that Daniel McCarthy 'had not been negligent', nor did they charge the Wellcome Foundation with 'general negligence'.[8] The basis of the complaint was that the system of manufacture at the Wellcome laboratory 'permitted sufficient negligence' to allow a bottle containing a suspension of tubercular bacilli to 'slip through their hands' and find its way into a bottle of TAF. Kelly asserted: 'in the same building within a few yards of each other were manufactured, health giving drugs and deadly poisons. Life and death were being manufactured side by side by Burroughs Wellcome, and the question would be, was the life sufficiently segregated from the death?'[9]

In response, J. M. Fitzgerald, denied that his clients the Wellcome Foundation had been negligent and explained that the preparations of tuberculin and the use of tubercle bacilli, occurred in premises isolated from those in which Wellcome manufactured other products. Fitzgerald asserted that his clients denied that they gave any warranty, that the children contracted tubercular disease as alleged, or that the preparation contained

---

5 *British Medical Journal* (5 June 1937), 1183.
6 Hansard, 'Diphtheria immunization', *Great Britain, Parliament, House of Commons*, Vol. 343, 46, cc. 1937–8W, 16 February 1939.
7 J. R. Hutchinson, Letter to R. P. McDonnell, 10 February 1939.
8 'Parents claim from chemists', *Irish Press*, 8 February 1939.
9 'Hearing opens in High Court of important action', *Cork Examiner*, 7 February 1939.

any poisonous or harmful ingredients. The defence suggested that McCarthy had simply been 'unlucky' enough to 'pick up a speck of tubercular sputum on a needle', or that he had 'struck a cold abscess containing tubercle' in the arm of one of the children treated, and 'unwittingly infected' the others.[10]

A series of medical witnesses including Dr Carney, private physician to the Cussen children, and Dr Fitzgerald and Dr O'Donovan of University College, Cork, gave evidence in support of Daniel McCarthy. All paid tribute to the 'high standard of routine and method' he employed.[11] Regarding defective sterilization, state pathologist Dr John McGrath, explained that tubercule bacilli, 'although relatively resistant to antiseptics, were easily killed by heat'. He stated his belief that the methods of sterilization employed at Dungarvan district hospital 'had been sufficient to kill any tubercle bacilli which may have been lodged in a syringe'. If dirty material remained on the swabs or syringe, he argued, they would have contained 'sore forming organisms' and no sores of that kind were found on the children. McGrath concluded that if the sore forming organisms had been killed 'then any tubercule bacilli would have been killed also'.[12]

Addressing the 'sputum' and 'cold abscess' theories as suggested by the defence, McGrath strenuously asserted that neither theory could explain events as they occurred at Ring. To substantiate the 'sputum' theory, McGrath argued that a person infected with tuberculosis would have had to be 'coughing out tubercle bacilli directly onto the syringe or needle', an occurrence that would have 'affected the next inoculated child in particular, and the rest of the children to a much lesser degree'. To infect all 24 children equally, he asserted that sputum would have to be 'spread uniformly in the antigen, and introduced in the bottle at the beginning of the inoculation session'.[13] Dr W. P. O'Callaghan, bacteriologist at Cork Street Fever Hospital, Dublin, also argued that the possibility of contamination arising from the syringe used by McCarthy was 'very remote'.[14]

Support for the 'cold abscess' theory required one of the children to have an abscess on their arm, a condition which generally presents only in a visibly sick child. McGrath claimed that in the unlikely event that McCarthy struck a cold abscess unwittingly: 'there would be no reason why the subsequent 23 children would have been infected equally'. Similarly, Dr William Boxwell, President of the Royal College of Physicians, testified that the position on the arm, where McCarthy gave inoculations, was not a likely

10 'Parents claim against drug firm', *Cork Examiner*, 8 February 1939.
11 'Inoculation methods at Ring College praised', *Cork Examiner*, 10 February 1939.
12 'Cork pathologist gives evidence in inoculation case', *Cork Examiner*, 11 February 1939.
13 *Cork Examiner*, 11 February 1939.
14 'Medical evidence in Ring College inoculation case', *Cork Examiner*, 14 February 1939.

place to find a cold abscess. Furthermore, Boxwell argued, in the 'extremely unlikely event' that McCarthy did push a needle through a cold abscess; he would not expect it to contain 'any appreciable concentration of tubercle bacilli, and certainly not enough to infect a further 23 children'.[15]

Counsel for the Wellcome Foundation, J. M. Fitzgerald, suggested that 'in Ireland there was a natural impulse to conceal consumption in a family'.[16] This line of defence was furthered by Fitzgerald's colleague Cecil Lavery who asserted that in Ireland, and particularly in rural areas, a large number of cases of pulmonary tuberculosis go undetected, 'with the death of a child being the first indication of tubercular infection in an elderly family member'.[17] Dr Dorothy Price, St Ultan's Hospital and consulting physician to the Royal National Hospital for Consumption, agreed that undetected cases of tuberculosis 'were not uncommon'. However, Price argued that the incidence of tuberculosis among children in Ireland was 'very much lower than in any other country yet reported on the continent of Europe'.[18] Price stated that she studied tuberculosis in children in Ireland and by applying the perculin skin test over several years she determined that less than 11 per cent of children aged 14 years, returned a positive reaction.[19]

Following eight days of testimony, the case for the plaintiffs closed. Counsel for Daniel McCarthy, Martin Maguire, applied for a direction in favour of his client, dismissing the action against him with costs, because there was no evidence of a contract between him and the plaintiffs for the sale of the material used by him in performing the inoculations. E. J. Kelly objected to the motion on the grounds that in addition to the contract to give professional services by inoculating the children, conjointly as part of his contract, McCarthy undertook to supply proper material: thereby 'implying warranty under the Sale of Goods Act, 1893'. Justice Maguire ruled that there was no evidence given of a contract of sale, and because the plaintiffs did not allege a charge of negligence against the doctor, he dismissed the action against McCarthy with costs.[20]

On 15 February, the defence evidence opened. In his opening remarks counsel for the Wellcome Foundation, J. M. Fitzgerald gave a brief history of Wellcome and stated that the not-for-profit foundation was set up in 1924 by Sir Henry Wellcome with the express intention of 'manufacturing medicaments for the alleviation of pain and suffering and the eradication of

15 *Cork Examiner*, 14 February 1939.
16 'Doctors evidence in High Court claim by parents', *Cork Examiner*, 9 February 1939.
17 *Cork Examiner*, 14 February 1939.
18 'Doctor dismissed from the Ring College action', *Cork Examiner*, 15 February 1939.
19 Dorothy Price, 'Tuberculosis in adolescents', *Irish Journal of Medical Science*, Vol. 14, No. 3 (1939), 124–29.
20 *Cork Examiner*, 15 February 1939.

disease'.[21] Fitzgerald conveyed the sense of 'tragedy' felt by those involved with the Wellcome Foundation that the plaintiffs alleged a charge of an 'extraordinary act of negligence' against them. He further stated that the allegation had 'sharply hit' the two principal officers at Wellcome, Richard O'Brien and Henry Parish, both of whom it was claimed 'were known to every medical man of standing as being two of the greatest contributors on the literature and the knowledge of the methods of healing diseases in children'. In sharp contrast, Fitzgerald charged that the plaintiffs had 'thrown the mantle of their protection around Dr McCarthy and in no way had his methods been complained of by them'. He continued: 'It is a misconception in law and a misconception in justice that he [McCarthy] should not have been made a defendant on the basis of the negligence that the plaintiffs charged against the Wellcome Foundation'.[22]

Fitzgerald stated that 'no part of the case depended on convicting McCarthy of any negligence', and insisted that he was not making the slightest charge against him. Instead, Fitzgerald asserted that he wanted to 'acquit Dr McCarthy of a very serious charge': 'that he used a bottle of tubercle bacilli and did not recognise it from a bottle of TAF', an occurrence, which would have let McCarthy open to a charge of serious neglect. In addition, Fitzgerald suggested that McCarthy was such a 'careless and happy go lucky gentleman' that he felt no compulsion to take a list of the children he was going to inoculate, and it was only 'a fortunate stroke of providence' that McCarthy did not find himself in serious trouble when the Cullen child was treated with TAF instead of APT.

Fitzgerald stated that if the bottle supplied by Wellcome contained tubercle bacilli instead of TAF the effect on the children would have been 'out of all comparison' to what transpired. Tubercle bacilli contain three billion bacilli in every cubic centimetre. Administration of such a 'dreadful mixture' to a child, would induce 'a severe reaction and a feverish sickness within 24 hours' and the child would be 'in a dying state' within a few weeks. In Ring, no child showed the slightest effects until a month after treatment. Fitzgerald argued that if the jury believed the evidence that Wellcome issued a bottle of tubercle bacilli then they must equally accept 'the scientific evidence of the ensuing reaction which the application of such a mixture would induce', a reaction that did not occur among children at Ring.[23]

Fitzgerald stated that staff at Wellcome manufactured TAF in a room as cut off from the room in which tubercle suspension was made 'as if there were

21 'Defence opened on behalf of drug manufacturers', *Cork Examiner*, 15 February 1939.
22 *Cork Examiner*, 15 February 1939.
23 *Cork Examiner*, 15 February 1939.

a sea between them' and he undertook to produce the 'senior hands in charge of the various departments' where filling, inspecting, counting, packing, and checking of serum was undertaken. Further to this, Fitzgerald asserted that he would rely on the 'truth and experience' of eminent pathologists to dispel any speculation regarding the 'minute care' taken in the production and testing of serum at Wellcome. In conclusion, Fitzgerald cautioned the jury: 'You can act neither on suspicion, surmise, or speculation. Acting on the true facts I say you must find that this charge of negligence has been made in the most extraordinary fashion and I believe quite recklessly and without one particle of real evidence to support it'.[24]

The first witness for the defence was Wellcome's principal bacteriologist, Henry Parish. He told the court that he was involved in the production of the anti-diphtheria prophylactic TAF since 1927 and that he was 'the first person to administer that antigen to a human subject'. Using a blackboard and easel in the court, Parish described in graphic detail how the prophylactic was prepared in the laboratory. He conceded that in the early stage of manufacture, the antigen contained toxin, 'which had been responsible for some severe reactions' in the past, however, he asserted that TAF manufactured by Wellcome was toxoid in which the harmful toxins had been killed, much like 'removing the fangs from a serpent'.

Parish described the series of elaborate tests that TAF underwent at Wellcome in compliance with the British Therapeutic Substances Act 1925. The first tested sterility 'to ensure that it contained no harmful organisms'. The second tested toxicity, which 'ensured the absence of poisons'. The third test was for potency to ensure that the preparation 'carried out the job it was intended for'. Finally, a purely chemical test ensured that 'the content of the preservative phenol was correct'.[25] Parish then produced record cards relating to two batches of TAF containing 13,000 doses from which the material used at Ring had come, and apart from the tragedy at Ring, Parish asserted that 'no complaint had been made as regards the toxicity of the serum and no serious symptoms had been reported'.[26]

Parish stated that having become aware of the Ring incident he visited Dungarvan on 6 March 1937 and saw some of the infected children at Ring College and at Dungarvan District Hospital. He agreed with the diagnosis that their lesions were tubercular. On securing a sample of unfinished TAF left over by Daniel McCarthy and bottles held by Michael O'Farrell, which came from the same batch, Parish conducted a series of tests to ascertain certain facts about the affair at Ring. He contested that the samples contained

24 *Cork Examiner*, 15 February 1939.
25 'Tragedy if immunization in Ireland suffers', *Cork Examiner*, 16 February 1939.
26 *Cork Examiner*, 16 February 1939.

no organisms and when injected into guinea pigs none showed evidence of tuberculosis. However, while investigating the effects of contact between an infected syringe and sterile TAF, Parish claimed that when a minute drop of tubercle-infected sputum was placed on the end of a syringe plunger, the sputum entered the bottle and infected the entire contents. Furthermore, Parish asserted that 'repeated experiments found that guinea pigs injected with 1 c.c. of infected TAF all developed tuberculosis'.[27]

During cross-examination, counsel for the plaintiffs, Brereton Barry, put it to Parish that the possibility that a fleck of sputum from an apparently uninfected person could get on a needle and then infect 24 children suggested that 'the immunization process itself was a highly dangerous activity'.[28] Barry referred to the Bundaberg disaster in Queensland where, he stated: 'a considerable amount of infection' occurred, and 12 children perished following anti-diphtheria immunization treatment. The defence were quick to clarify that the serum used at Bundaberg was manufactured by the Commonwealth State Laboratories and not by the Wellcome Foundation, and that the real significance of the Bundaberg incident was 'that it drew a parallel with the incident at Ring in that in both cases the serum had become contaminated by accident or negligence'.[29]

In defence of the anti-diphtheria immunization process, and in support of the Wellcome Foundation, Dr Jack Saunders testified that in the years 1929–38, he and the Cork public health department administered almost 35,000 injections of anti-diphtheria serum without incident, and that 'they had used nothing else but the products of the Wellcome Research Laboratories'.[30] Similarly, Dr Christopher McSweeney stated that he immunized 'around 10,000 children against diphtheria using Wellcome products' in Dublin and in his opinion 'TAF was the most reliable prophylactic available'. Both Saunders and McSweeney were strong advocates of anti-diphtheria immunization and they echoed sentiments expressed by Henry Parish when he stated 'I would hate to think that because of this disaster, immunization would suffer in Ireland. That would be a tragedy of the first order'.[31]

Throughout the hearing, the courtroom was crowded every day, and the level of interest displayed in the case was evident by the column inches devoted to chronicling every epee and parry. In the *Irish Press* Anna Kelly described the scene thus:

27 *Cork Examiner*, 16 February 1939.
28 'Expert tells of vital tests in inoculation case', *Irish Times*, 16 February 1939.
29 'Court told of Queensland disaster', *Irish Times*, 22 February 1939. See also, C. Hooker, 'Diphtheria, immunization and the Bundaberg tragedy'.
30 *Irish Times*, 22 February 1939.
31 *Irish Times*, 16 February 1939.

The court is crowded and thick with wigs fore and aft [...] It is a very intent and attentive court, for this is the case of the century. A case unparalleled in law, the case of Ring College, the Battle of the Bacilli. Doctors and lawyers pitting their best wits [...] They sit together in amity, but jump up in acrimony. There is tragedy behind this case and big issues before it [...] The jury listened intensely to the legal symphony. Quiet, passionate, thrilling.[32]

On 23 February 1939, evidence concluded and the president, Justice Maguire, intimated that he would 'let the case go to the jury'. Cecil Lavery, counsel for the defence told the jury that they had to discharge 'possibly the heaviest burden that had ever fallen to the lot of a jury in this country'.[33] He asked the jury not to consider the fact that the immunization system saved the lives of 'tens of thousands of children', and although everyone who had knowledge of the case must feel 'the keenest sympathy' with the O'Cionnfaola family, he asserted that the jury should not be swayed unduly by 'sympathy which the situation of the plaintiff aroused'.[34]

Counsel for the plaintiffs, Brereton Barry told the jury that every line of inquiry was tried at Ring to solve this 'mystery of science', but it was only when they had gone to the Wellcome laboratories in Beckenham that they at last found 'masses of infection' in the form of live tubercle bacilli. He asserted that it would be a terrible message for the world if it were to go out from the court that the system employed by the Wellcome laboratories was such that 'a bottle containing deadly poison could come out of their works, and that they were powerless to prevent it. This great firm cannot take up that attitude'.[35]

In his summing up, Justice Maguire reiterated the seriousness and importance of this 'sensational' case and that 'upon him and the jury rested a very heavy responsibility'[36]. He stated:

If the evidence leaves you in doubt between two possibilities–one, that the infection came from the bottle as it came from Beckenham, or, the other, that it came from the bottle infected by something that happened while it was in Dr McCarthy's hands–if you cannot make up your minds between these two alternatives, then the plaintiffs fail.[37]

32 Anna Kelly, 'Around the town', *Irish Press*, 23 February 1939.
33 'Evidence concluded in Ring inoculation case', *Irish Times*, 23 February 1939.
34 *Irish Times*, 23 February 1939.
35 *Irish Times*, 23 February 1939.
36 'Verdict for chemist in Ring College case', *Irish Times*, 24 February 1939.
37 *Irish Times*, 24 February 1939.

Justice Maguire questioned whether it was necessary to ask a jury of 'intelligent Irish men' to put out of their minds 'any prejudice as between Irish plaintiffs and English defendants' and directed them to deliberate on one question only. Did the defendants, the Wellcome Foundation Ltd., negligently issue a bottle containing live tubercle bacilli in a suspension for use instead of a bottle of TAF? [38] After an absence of 25 minutes, the jury returned an answer of 'no', and gave judgement for the defendants with costs.

The High Court proceedings brought no solace for the grieving O'Cionnfaola family, and the inconclusive verdict, which exonerated the attending physician Daniel McCarthy, and failed to uphold the charge levelled against the Wellcome Foundation, undermined public confidence in active immunization to the extent that numbers presenting for treatment fell by more than 80 per cent. The Ring College immunization disaster was a tragic and disturbing case, which attracted huge public and professional attention, all caught up in the profound and very public disagreement between the local physician Dr Daniel McCarthy and the suppliers of the anti-diphtheria vaccine, the Wellcome Foundation Ltd. In a landmark High Court case, the jury failed to apportion blame to either party, thereby dealing a serious blow to established immunization schemes in Ireland, and a fatal blow to calls for a government backed immunization scheme in Britain.

After Ring

By the end of 1936, the Irish Free State was at the cusp of establishing a national anti-diphtheria immunization programme. This is a noteworthy achievement. State-backed anti-diphtheria programmes did not make ground in mainland Europe until 1938, and pursued with any vigour only when wartime conditions forced the issue from 1941 onwards.[39] If the Irish immunization programme progressed unimpeded, it seemed destined to exert complete control over diphtheria, and to become the first established national childhood immunization programme in Europe. However, the death of Siobhán O'Cionnfaola, and the subsequent controversy surrounding the Ring incident, asked serious questions of active immunization and

38 *Irish Times*, 24 February 1939.
39 See Jane Lewis, 'The prevention of diphtheria in Canada and Britain, 1914–45', *Journal of Social History*, Vol. 20 (1986), 163–76. See also, Beyazova and Yucel, 'Age specific diphtheria immunity', in Ben S. Wheeler (ed.), Trends in diphtheria research (New York, 2006), 119–34, and also, European Centre for Disease 'A historical perspective', *Prevention and Control, Scientific panel on childhood immunization schedule: Diphtheria-tetanus-pertussis (DTP) vaccination.* http://www.ecdc.europa.eu/en/publications/Publications/0911_GUI_Scientific_Panel_on_Childhood_Immunization_DTP.pdf.

undermined vaccine confidence among parents, doctors and politicians. It is remarkable that the health inspector for Dungarvan, Dr J. D. Hourihane failed to acknowledge the tragedy at Ring in his reports and official DLG&PH publications make no mention of the episode. However, the incident did force Minister O'Kelly and his department to reconsider existing legislation designed to control the quality of therapeutic substances used in the state.

Although Free State health authorities introduced the Therapeutic Substances Act in 1932, the legislation limited the remit of the associated advisory board to the evaluation of catgut, and various other veterinary products.[40] The Ring incident was a wakeup call for Minister O'Kelly. He appointed a new advisory committee, under the guidance of Professor O'Kelly, UCD, to assist in making orders and regulations concerning the strength, quality, and purity of substances covered by the Act; the tests used for determining if the required standards were attained, and units of standardization.[41] Prior to the introduction of the Therapeutic Substances Act, the chief safeguard ensuring the quality of imported serums was reliance on the producer of the goods, and 'the very natural desire of the manufacturer to see that his product maintained a good reputation and that accidents did not occur following their administration'. In this regard, the safety or otherwise of serums used in Ireland relied solely on the honour of the manufacturer, as the licensing authority in England was under no obligation to test samples of batches for export, and did not do so unless a complaint arose.[42] Peculiarly, Professor O'Kelly had highlighted the shortcomings of this system in November 1936, the same month in which children at Ring College received treatment. At that time, the DLG&PH ignored his concerns. Six months later, when the Ring incident became public, the department conceded previous 'safeguards' had been insufficient.

Fatalities due to excessive toxicity of therapeutic substances were known to occur; but were rare occurrences in the Free State. The area that caused most concern for medical practitioners did not relate to undue toxicity of imported serums, but to their 'very variable', or 'uniformly low potency'. One concern was that foreign manufacturers had 'a great opportunity of making profit' by reducing the strength of their preparations so that more of the product would be required. Another concern was that a firm might produce a substandard product 'not having the requisite plant, or the technical advice requisite to enable them to produce preparations of high potency'. These were the most common concerns voiced by doctors concerning imported serums.

40 NAI, HLTH/B1/38/41, W. D. O' Kelly, Letter to R. P. McDonnell DLG&PH, 30 October 1936.
41 DLG&PH, *Report 1936–37*, 134. *Therapeutic Substances Act*, 1932–*Advisory Committee*.
42 DLG&PH, *Report 1932–33*, 100.

Complaints from general practitioners regarding the variable standard of imported products usually took the line that 'one firms diphtheria antitoxin was no use, that another's Salvarsan was the best, and that other vaccines were useless'. While acknowledging that some observations may have been prompted by the suggestions of salesmen representing one or other pharmaceutical company, central health conceded that such statements were made so frequently that 'there would appear that some real foundation for the suspicion that the products under discussion varied as regard their potency'.[43]

Minister O'Kelly and his department acknowledged that the manufacture and importation of therapeutic substances in Great Britain, Europe, and North America was under state control in those districts, and that 'the public and the medical practitioner alike look to the State to ensure the trustworthiness of these articles when offered for sale'. With the exception of vaccine lymph, and stock vaccines, the manufacture of therapeutic substances in the Free State was not extensive, and the bulk of substances in use were imports. Diphtheria antitoxin alone was imported by seven different manufacturers: Sharpe and Dohme, Philadelphia; Boroughs and Wellcome, London; Evans and Sons, Liverpool; Bayer Products Ltd, Germany; Eli Lilly and Co, London; The Lister Institute, Hertfordshire; and the Connaught Laboratories, Canada.[44]

Professor O'Kelly intimated that he was amenable to act as inspector under Section 16 of the Therapeutic Substances Act and he was prepared to undertake 'a certain amount of testing in the case of diphtheria antitoxin and diphtheria prophylactics' if samples could be collected by 'a responsible person' acting on behalf of the inspector. This position subsequently filled by S. G. O'Neill, a pharmacist in the employ of the DLG&PH, ensured that O'Kelly received samples of diphtheria antitoxin directly from the place of manufacture, from an importer, or from premises where a holder of a research licence kept the item.[45] In addition, in his capacity as inspector under the Therapeutic Substances Act, O'Kelly was entitled to enter and inspect premises, plant, process of manufacture, and the means employed to standardize and test therapeutic substances. During 1937, he inspected 13 pharmaceutical companies in Britain and France. In October the same year, O'Kelly attended an inter-governmental conference on biological standardization in Geneva, where representatives agreed that international standards adopted by the Permanent Commission on Biological Standardisation of the Health Organisation 'should be made effective by the competent authorities

43 DLG&PH, *Report 1932–33*, 100.
44 NAI, HLTH/B1/38/41.
45 NAI, HLTH/B1/38/41, Seán T. O'Kelly, Letter to R. P. McDonnell, 9 November 1936.

of all countries'. While Free State health authorities agreed to adopt international standards recommended by the Commission, the DLG&PH resolved that therapeutic substances imported from outside the state would continue to be standardized against regulations in the country of manufacture, as recommended by the League of Nations.[46]

Central health remained adamant that anti-diphtheria immunization was 'our best weapon' against diphtheria. However, wide media coverage, and great public interest in the Ring controversy, and the speculative nature of its causation, had seriously undermined confidence in active immunization. Between 1936 and 1939, attendance at established schemes declined by more than 80 per cent; falling from 2,199 to 442 in Cork, and from 30,934 to 6,177 in Dublin over the corresponding period.[47] Low attendances forced a temporary cessation of immunization in many districts and medical officers in County Cavan, Laois, Longford, Louth, and Monaghan abandoned their schemes completely. Although J. D. Hourihane reported that immunization continued in districts under his control, participation had been 'disappointing'. In the northern health district, P. R. Fanning reported that the immunization schemes in operation in districts under his control remained inadequate, and largely under-subscribed.[48] The reduced number of children presented for immunization treatment during 1938 reversed the downward trend in incidence recorded in previous years. Almost 3,000 diphtheria cases occurred, up from 2,511 the previous year: an increase of 15 per cent. Central Health regarded this as an unwelcome development and remained convinced that increased prevalence correlated directly with 'the intensive propaganda that has been carried out recently against immunization by opponents of the practice, which has delayed the production of herd immunity'.[49]

In November 1938, Cashel Urban Council debated the introduction of an anti-diphtheria immunization scheme as suggested by local medical officer Dr Naughton. Naughton cautioned that 'diphtheria of fatal character was present in the town'.[50] Councillor Michael Davern remonstrated that people had 'bitter memories of 1936 [...] and the Ring affair' and that Naughton would find little support for his motion.[51] Davern claimed that Italy and Austria turned down immunization schemes because of 'serious reactions to

46 DLG&PH, *Report 1937–38*, 122.
47 J. C. Saunders, *Annual report of the Medical Officer of Health for Cork County Borough* (Cork, 1939), 15. Also, M. J. Russell, *Report of the State of Public Health in the City of Dublin for the two years ending 31 December 1940* (Dublin, 1941), 41.
48 DLG&PH, *Report 1937–38*, 165–73.
49 DLG&PH, *Report 1938–39*, 30.
50 'Councillors "No" to MOH', *Irish Independent*, 5 November 1938.
51 'Council rejects immunization scheme', *Irish Press*, 5 November 1938.

immunization serums' and he claimed personal knowledge of eight children in his own district being 'done slowly to death' as a result of anti-diphtheria immunization treatment.[52] Mrs M. Davern, whose children Treasa and Eugene fell ill after inoculation at Ring College, stressed that in light of the events at Ring, the proposal to introduce immunization in Cashel 'was an outlandish proposal'. Addressing Cashel council Mrs Davern exclaimed 'You all know what happened to my little girl. I took her to the best doctors. This has meant for me two years of suffering and worry. I for one would not approve of the immunization scheme. I would not like to hear of another disaster'.[53] On Councillor Davern's recommendation, and following Mrs Davern's plea, the council rejected the motion to introduce immunization in Cashel. Furthermore, councillors agreed to erect hoardings in the town to warn parents against 'the alleged dangers of permitting their children to be inoculated against diphtheria'.[54] Similarly, in March 1939, Dr O'Riely, county medical officer for Cavan, lamented that although a diphtheria scheme 'was badly needed in the county' public interest in the Ring case 'would prevent any voluntary scheme being carried through with success at present'.[55]

To complicate things even further, members of the Irish Medical Union hijacked the tragedy at Ring to support demands for increased fees for immunization services. This demand formed the basis of a pre-existing dispute between the DLG&PH and the Irish Free State Medical Union whose membership represented 80 per cent of medical practitioners in the state. The agreed fee in place in 1936 was 1/6d per case, however, doctors insisted on an increased minimum fee of 3/6d per case, or, £2.2.0 per session of twelve cases.[56] Staying true to form, a frugal Minister O'Kelly refused the doctors' demands. In response, union secretary Dr Michael Casey, instructed members to withdraw immunization services on the basis that 'the extra amount to be earned by each doctor is very small indeed and it is not the amount that is our deep concern but the principle involved in the case'.[57]

In the wake of the Ring College immunization accident, the medical union became less concerned with fees and voiced new concerns relating to the indemnity of their members, particularly with regard to complaints arising from complications caused by immunizing serum supplied to them. In December 1938, secretary to the County Galway Medical Doctors' Association, Dr O'Leary, inquired as to what precautions the local health

52 *Irish Press*, 5 November 1938.
53 'Council rejects immunization', *Munster Express*, 11 November 1938.
54 *Irish Press*, 5 November 1938.
55 *Anglo-Celt*, 4 March 1939.
56 NAI HLTH/B29/24. File on the Ring Immunization Disaster 1935–48.
57 File on the Ring Immunization Disaster 1935–48.

board were taking to indemnify doctors against such complaints, and quoted the 'unfortunate case in Ring' as an example.[58] Doctors suspended anti-diphtheria immunization in County Mayo on similar grounds.[59] As no agreement on indemnity, or remuneration ensued, medical union members withdrew their anti-diphtheria services leaving many Irish children without preventive, or curative, protection against diphtheria.[60]

The medical union's decision to withdraw services left established immunization schemes in a precarious position. Boards of health could only pay fees sanctioned by the Minister; however, it was the duty of every board to safeguard child health in their districts. Addressing the matter in Dublin, board of health member Mr Rollins stated that 'doctors had a right to strike if they liked'. However, he asked 'Were they to endanger the lives of little children, and perhaps see many of them in their coffins, while the doctors and the Minister argue about fees?'[61] Many general practitioners shared Rollin's sentiments. While desperate to implement immunization schemes that many fought to get sanctioned, doctors could not deviate from union 'strike action' without damaging their professional standing. In County Clare, local medical officer Dr G. P. McCarthy stated:

It is rather hellish to me to see this scheme not being implemented. The board did its share, yet the scheme is now held up as a result of a dispute over fees [...] the fatality of the whole thing was seeing children dying for lack of immunization.[62]

Faced with an outbreak of diphtheria in the Mountshannon area of County Clare, and an accompanying demand from parents in the district for an intervention, McCarthy contacted the medical union to suggest that he might implement an emergency immunization scheme there. The union adamantly refused McCarthy's request unless the Minister sanctioned higher fees for the work. McCarthy resolved that as the board of health had sanctioned immunization in County Clare, it was his duty to intervene, and immunized 480 children without fees, pending settlement of the dispute. McCarthy gained the support of fellow practitioners' Dr W. Shannon of Carrigaholt, and Dr Mary Courtney of Killaloe, who also agreed to carry out immunization work without fees.[63] However, due to suspected interference

---

58 *Tuam Herald*, 24 December 1938.
59 'County Mayo Health Bill', *Connaught Telegraph*, 8 July 1939.
60 Local disputes relating to indemnity appear in the *Tuam Herald*, 24 December 1938, and the *Connaught Telegraph*, 8 July 1939.
61 'Doctors on strike', *Irish Times*, 6 October 1937.
62 'Doctors to work without fees', *Irish Times*, 2 March 1938.
63 *Irish Times*, 2 March 1938.

by the medical union, Drs Shannon, and Courtney subsequently rescinded their offer.

As no other general practitioner or dispensary doctor would act against the medical union and assist McCarthy, the board of health sought to overcome the difficulty by appointing a temporary Immunization Officer at a rate of £10 10s per week. The board took the decision on the basis that Dublin health authorities had employed a temporary 'medical immuniser' without the approval of the medical union, but without protest from them either.[64] In October 1938, the Clare board of health sanctioned Dr Patricia Milligan to take up a similar position in County Clare. Over the course of three weeks, Milligan administered an initial dose of anti-diphtheria antigen to 3,000 children.[65] These numbers suggest that Milligan undertook her duty in a zealous manner; however, she resigned from the position after just three weeks quoting 'the attitude of the Irish Medical Union and its Clare Branch' for her decision. A letter from Milligan, read before a meeting of the board of health meeting in Ennis, stated that 'much correspondence' from the Irish Medical Union had made it 'perfectly clear' to her that her appointment as Immunization Officer, and all similar appointments 'were now very definitely banned'. Milligan stated:

> My tenure of the position during the interim period was both uncomfortable and invidious, but whatever my inclinations were, I felt it a duty to the board to take up and carry out the duties of the appointment until the status of the office in the eyes of the profession was made perfectly clear. That has now been done, and the Irish Medical Union has registered its disapproval to me in no uncertain terms, So, I beg to tender my resignation to the board.[66]

Health board chairman, Mr J. Fahy, stated that, as far as the health of Clare children was concerned, the threats made against Dr Milligan were a very serious matter. Three children died of diphtheria the week before Milligan's appointment and one board member, Mr O'Loughlin, charged:

> We are responsible before God for seeing that this matter of the deaths of three children is fully investigated and those responsible brought to book. These children were really murdered as a result of not being immunised.

64 'Union explains doctor's stand', *Irish Independent*, 3 November 1938.
65 'Clare doctor's praise for immunization', *Irish Times*, 16 November 1938.
66 'Doctors blamed for deaths', *Irish Times*, 26 October 1938.

Dr McCarthy remarked that if the board were to 'take dictation of the kind now indulged in' it would 'paralyse' health services in the county. McCarthy intimated that he wrote to doctors throughout County Clare to elicit participation in an emergency immunization scheme and many expressed willingness to do so. However, all subsequently withdrew support claiming 'a good deal behind this opposition to the scheme'. He suggested that the Board should probe such 'sinister opposition' to the last. An exasperated McCarthy exclaimed:

> It is time that this thing was stopped, and stopped with venom, not with any sugar-stick action. I am fed up with it. These people are crying out for immunization for their children, and what the devil can we do? The board has provided the immunization material and we are paralysed. I think it is a scandal, and I never heard of a situation like it in all my existence. It means the lives of the children of County Clare versus a bob.[67]

Media coverage of the Milligan affair did not show the medical union in a good light; and a letter to the *Irish Times* from the union secretary, J. C. Martin did little to rectify the matter. Martin argued that while the union 'strongly encouraged' immunization schemes, responsibility for their implementation lay with the DLG&PH and county health boards. Martin suggested that many health boards were willing to pay 'reasonable remuneration' but were 'held in check' by Minister O'Kelly.[68] Furthermore, Martin asserted that the union had always approved of immunization 'when there was any pressing need' and the union would not object to immunization treatment in any district where 'an emergency' might arise. Martin asserted that if Dr McCarthy had made the union aware of the high incidence of disease in County Clare 'he could have had the cordial co-operation of the medical profession in his campaign'.[69]

At an emergency meeting to discuss Dr Milligan's resignation, a representative of the Clare branch of the medical union, J. F. McNamara, stated that the union regarded Milligan's appointment as 'annoying' because it appeared to them 'to be aimed at breaking the power of the medical union in the country'. He claimed that Milligan's appointment was 'unnecessary and vexatious, and calculated to undermine the influence of the medical union in Clare'.[70] McNamara admitted that members of the union had

67 *Irish Times*, 26 October 1938.
68 'Letter to the editor: Immunization', *Irish Times*, 28 October 1938.
69 *Irish Times*, 28 October 1938.
70 'Medical Union's attitude', *Irish Times*, 2 November 1938.

refused to carry out routine immunization in Clare 'because they should receive the same remuneration as medical professionals in the North', and he further asserted that all union members were 'ready and willing' to immunize against diphtheria 'if an urgent necessity for such immunization was considered to exist'. However, he argued that the union 'had never been led to believe that the board were duly alarmed over the question of diphtheria immunization in Clare'.[71]

In essence, the medical union were willing to intervene only in cases where increased prevalence of diphtheria forced a medical officer to declare a 'state of emergency' in their district. This stance was little more than a sideswipe at county medical officers as a cohort. In many districts, newly appointed medical officers encountered sustained opposition from local general practitioners concerned with issues relating to medical authority and traditional revenue streams. Clare was the last county in the Free State to appoint a full-time county medical officer, and did so only because of sustained ministerial pressure to do so. It is likely that opposition to McCarthy's appointment as medical officer underscored the staunch non-cooperative stance maintained by the Clare branch of the medical union against childhood immunization.

In their bid to undermine medical officers as a cohort, the medical union also sought to discredit the immunization process itself. During a health board meeting in Ennis, union representative McNamara claimed their members 'regarded immunization as still being in the experimental stage'. Invoking Ring, he stated that 'doctors were well aware of the fact that some very regrettable incidents occurred as a result of immunization [...] and that doctors could not guarantee that immunization against diphtheria would be effective in any particular case'. Subsequently, rumours circulated throughout County Clare that 'stuff had been sent around the county' and that persons immunized with it 'become violently ill'. Dr McCarthy publicly stated his belief that these rumours emanated from the Clare branch of the medical union, and that there was 'no substantiation for any such allegations'. He further asserted that 'the circulation of such rumours was a very poisonous propaganda and most unfair'.[72] The medical union dismissed McCarthy's assertion stating they 'resented such an accusation' and that as a 'responsible medical body', they 'never cavilled against the efficacy of the scheme' and had 'always been most anxious to have immunization done'.[73] Minister O'Kelly appealed to members of the medical union to reconsider their stance. He asserted that the success of the anti-diphtheria campaign

71 *Irish Times*, 2 November 1938.
72 'Poison propaganda denounced', *Irish Times*, 16 November 1938.
73 'New turn in Clare dispute', *Irish Times*, 14 December 1938.

depended on the 'loyal cooperation' of the medical profession, as responsibility for recognizing diphtheria and administering antitoxin at an early stage rested with them. Furthermore, he stressed the importance of the cooperation of medical practitioners if the full value of preventive measures were to be realized. O'Kelly bemoaned the 'unfortunate dispute regarding fees', however, he acknowledged that many practitioners 'carried on the good work without fee or reward'.[74] The minister 'earnestly hoped' for a settlement during 1938, however, the dispute rumbled on for a further ten years; the medical union refusing to implement anti-diphtheria immunization until health minister Noel Browne capitulated to union demands for increased fees, which settled the matter in 1948.

74 Department of Local Government and Public Health, *Report 1939–40* (Dublin Stationery Office, 1940), 33.

7

Towards a
National Immunization Programme

ight diphtheria related fatalities recorded in Cork city during 1936 brought the total number of such fatalities recorded in the city over the previous four years to 192. Notably, in every child fatality, none had presented for preventive treatment. Of 14,210 children presented for treatment, not one died from diphtheria, even though they endured continuous exposure to an intensive and virulent form of infection.[1] These results attracted both national and international attention, and received positive coverage in the *Proceedings of the Royal Society of Medicine* in July 1936. The article, submitted by Professor John McLeod of Leeds, confirmed that incidence of diphtheria in Cork city for the twenty-five years to 1936 was 'one of the highest or absolutely the highest ever recorded in any area [...] and three times as high as the worst areas in England and Wales'.[2] Referring to the marked decline in the incidence of diphtheria in Cork, McLeod asserted that the very large proportion of the child population treated may have played a significant part in the decline of diphtheria in the city, which he claimed 'is today the most completely immunised in Europe'.[3]

In his comprehensive study of anti-diphtheria immunization in England, Wales, Scotland, and Ireland during the years 1929–36, Graham Forbes bolstered McLeod's claims regarding the immunological position of Cork city. Forbes found that, taken as a whole, anti-diphtheria schemes in England, Wales, and Scotland achieved immunization rates representing an average of 5 per cent of the total population, and 22 per cent of the child population.[4]

---

1 CCCLS/352.4. Saunders, *Report of the Medical Officer of Health for the year 1935*, 14–15.
2 John McLeod, *Proceedings of the Royal Society of Medicine*, Vol. XXIX (July 1936), section on pathology.
3 McLeod, *Proceedings of the Royal Society of Medicine*, July 1936.
4 J. Graham Forbes, 'Progress of diphtheria prevention; a survey and some results', *British Medical Journal* (18 December 1937), 1209.

Forbes highlighted the extraordinary reduction in incidence and mortality achieved in New York and Montreal, major urban centres that achieved immunization rates of 65 per cent, and 50 per cent respectively, amongst their respective child populations. With regard to Britain and Ireland, Forbes found that Cork city alone achieved immunization rates comparable with North America and Canada, accounting for 15 per cent of the total population and 53 per cent of the child population.[5]

More importantly, the high rate of immunity achieved in Cork effected a 96 per cent reduction in diphtheria morbidity and an 87 per cent reduction in diphtheria mortality there. Nationally, a 10 per cent reduction in diphtheria mortality coincided with the rollout of anti-diphtheria immunization in the years 1930–36; however, if we consider that diphtheria morbidity in the Free State increased by over 56 per cent over the corresponding period then Jack Saunders's achievement in Cork was nothing short of astonishing. Despite the continuing dispute between the DLG&PH and the Irish Medical Union regarding immunization fees, and the continuing reticence of a sizeable proportion of parents to subject their children to immunization treatment, Saunders's perseverance brought the prospect of a diphtheria-free city close to realization; the Ring College disaster and the death of Siobhán O'Cionnfaola dashed any hopes of achieving this.

The first six months of 1937 registered some of the lowest attendances recorded at the Cork immunization clinic. A short, sharp outbreak of diphtheria, which claimed the lives of 17 children in the city during the summer, compelled some parents to present their children for treatment; however, for the whole of 1937 the number of children presented fell by 50 per cent on the previous year.[6] The falloff in attendance upset the delicate balancing act of maintaining herd immunity, and somewhat expectedly, diphtheria cases rose substantially. Eighty cases occurred during 1937, up from 25 the previous year. Seventeen fatalities ensued, maintaining a relatively high case fatality rate of 21.2 per cent. The consistently high fatality rate suggested that if a child in Cork city contracted diphtheria, the chances for survival were little over one in four, and the factors underpinning these statistics showed no sign of abating. The diphtheria strain prevalent in the city maintained an exceptionally virulent character. The growing proportion of parents reluctant to present children for treatment facilitated increased incidence. Prolonged delay in seeking medical advice was common and parents of at least four diphtheria fatalities recorded during 1937 had refused immunization treatment for their children. In two separate cases,

---

5 Forbes, *British Medical Journal* (1937), 1212.
6 CCCLS/352.4. J. C. Saunders, *Report of the Medical Officer of Health for the year 1937*, 18.

parents sought medical attention after an interval of seven days, and in one case, a delay of four days ensued.[7]

A deviation from the characteristic dispersion of diphtheria occurred during 1937, in the sense that incidence in children aged two years and under fell significantly. This may have been due to a decision in early 1936 to extend immunization services to include infants (aged one year and under). In 1937, most fatalities occurred in the four to six age group, and one death occurred in a woman aged 34 years. Although this is an unusual feature of diphtheria, Saunders confirmed that this woman was in contact with a definite case of diphtheria and delayed treatment for five days, with fatal results.[8] Increased diphtheria cases in Cork during 1937 mirrored a pan-European recrudescence of the disease.[9] Notwithstanding this, in 1938 incidence in the city decreased to 54 cases, and the resultant seven fatalities, and fatality rate of 12.7 per cent, was one of the lowest on record. Again, none of the child fatalities had received any form of anti-diphtheria treatment. Saunders lamented that these deaths were not only preventable, but also constituted 'a blot on our record'. Facilities for protecting children against diphtheria had been available in the city for almost ten years, and Saunders laid the blame for the child deaths 'entirely upon the shoulders of those parents who neglect to avail of them'.[10]

However, the relatively low morbidity and mortality rates induced a false sense of security among parents and affected a further diminution in the number of children presented for immunization treatment. This trend continued during 1939 when only 355 children completed the full course of treatment. Despite this, incidence maintained a downward trend during 1939, with 41 notified cases, and three fatalities, maintaining a low case fatality rate of 7.4 per cent.[11] A slight rise in diphtheria morbidity and mortality occurred during 1940. Fifty-two cases notified and five fatalities ensued. Attendance at the municipal immunization clinic remained low, and as a result, the proportion of the child population left without immunity to diphtheria steadily increased. Saunders worried that the reappearance of diphtheria in epidemic form became an increasingly likely prospect and a possible shortage of antitoxin due to war conditions did little to quell his concerns.[12]

7 Saunders, *Report 1937*, 15.
8 Saunders, *Report 1937*, 15.
9 *Statistical Department of the Health Section of the League of Nations*, as quoted in Saunders, *Report 1937*, 16.
10 CCCLS/352.4. J. C. Saunders, *Report of the Medical Officer of Health for the year 1938*, 13.
11 CCCLS/352.4. J. C. Saunders, *Report of the Medical Officer of Health for the year 1939*, 13.
12 CCCLS/352.4. J. C. Saunders, *Report of the Medical Officer of Health for the year 1940*, 9.

Sixty-two cases notified during 1941 and five fatalities ensued. Three fatalities occurred in untreated children aged six years and under, though the remaining two fatalities again occurred in adult women, aged 60 and 38 years. Another notable occurrence during 1941 was that no diphtheria fatality occurred in the six to fifteen age group: a group on whom the ill effects of diphtheria characteristically fell heaviest. It would seem that immunization successfully protected children of school-going age, but pushed incidence outside its traditional sphere to affect pre-school and adult populations. By 1941, the scheme for voluntary immunization against diphtheria had been available in Cork city for 13 years. During that time, 17,915 children received full immunization treatment and not a single fatality occurred among this group. In the same period, diphtheria claimed the lives of 223 unimmunized children. Again, Saunders blamed these fatalities 'entirely on parents who have been so negligent as to not avail of facilities for protection against diphtheria'. As far as he was concerned, apart from putting their own children at risk, growing numbers of non-immunized children threatened to diminish the 'herd immunity' of the community as a whole, and as happened so often in the past, led to a distinct tendency towards increased incidence, and increased fatalities.[13]

In 1942, the city experienced another major diphtheria epidemic, registering a rate of incidence not seen since 1929. Saunders reported:

> While it was obvious that a major epidemic would make its appearance sooner or later, taking into consideration the prevalent indifference to immunization, there was no reason to suspect that it would commence so soon or that it would spread so rapidly as the disease did during the past year. Parents and the public generally have been warned again and again both in these Reports and in the public press of the consequences of neglect in the protection of their children, notwithstanding such warnings the great majority of them continued indifferent, with the consequences we now know. The epidemic which is now reported may not have been as large or as virulent as some of those reported in former years but, nevertheless, it has been of definitely major dimensions.[14]

January 1942 was marked by a marginal increase in the incidence of diphtheria in the city, averaging two to three cases per week. However, in February, 27

13 CCCLS/352.4. J. C. Saunders, *Report of the Medical Officer of Health for the year 1941*, 21.
14 CCCLS/352.4. J. C. Saunders, *Report of the Medical Officer of Health for the year 1942*, 14.

cases notified and 'ushered in the epidemic proper'. Incidence increased month on month, peaking in October, when 61 cases notified in that month alone. By the end of the year, 372 cases occurred in the city: a 600 per cent increase on the average number of cases recorded for the five years previously. Incidence among adolescents and adults showed a marked increase, accounting for 15 per cent of total cases. However, incidence again fell heaviest on children of school-going age representing 57 per cent of all reported cases. Of the ensuing 21 fatalities, all were children aged ten years and under.[15]

Analysis of diphtheria cases recorded in 1942 reveals that July, August, and December showed a definite decrease in cases, those periods corresponding directly with school closures for summer and Christmas holidays. This being so, it seems clear that schools continued to play a predominant role in propagating the disease, and probably in initiating the outbreak. Early in the year, a number of cases occurred in a school on the north side of the city. On investigation, the public health department found that every case reported in the school came from one classroom. Throat swabs taken from 85 children attending the school revealed that almost 10 per cent of the school population were diphtheria 'carriers'. When these 'carriers' were subsequently removed from the school and quarantined, diphtheria cases recorded among students attending this particular school returned to normal levels. In June 1942, a similar sharp spike in incidence occurred in a school on the south side of the city. This area, regarded as 'the best immunised area in the city' had, apart from isolated incidents, managed to remain clear of diphtheria. An investigation revealed that all cases again came from one classroom, and of the 54 children subjected to throat swabbing, 14 children, or 26 per cent of the student population there were identified as 'carriers'.

Overcrowded classrooms, combined with defective ventilation, were major factors in the rapid spread of diphtheria among schoolchildren. While these conditions were universal in city schools, conditions at the south side school were more acute. Although children attended lessons in a newly erected building, ongoing structural alterations in older school buildings meant that children endured severe overcrowding for prolonged periods during the school day.[16] As a precautionary measure, the public health department closed down the entire infant department, a measure that immediately terminated the epidemic in this particular school. Highlighting the fact that during school life, 'children are most exposed to the risks of the more dangerous infectious diseases', Saunders asserted that there was 'a moral obligation on the state to see that their environment while at school is as free from such danger as it is possible to effect by human agency'.

15 Saunders, *Report 1942*, 21.
16 Saunders, *Report 1942*, 18.

The use of throat swabs to identify diphtheria 'carriers' played an important role in arresting outbreaks of diphtheria in city schools. The identification and quarantine of diphtheria 'carriers' proved to be an effective intervention, particularly when the disease appeared in epidemic form. In 1942, the public health department subjected 3,500 schoolchildren to throat swabbing, incurring a cost of £670 on the municipal authority. Saunders considered the high cost of laboratory services utilized to process throat swabs as a serious drawback to efforts to control diphtheria during periods of epidemicity. He appealed to laboratory authorities at UCC requesting a reduction in charges, 'due to the exceptional circumstances prevailing in the city'.[17] It may have been that chief bacteriologist at UCC, William O'Donovan, held some resentment towards Saunders following their differing stances on the Ring College affair, or O'Donovan may have made his decision based solely on fiscal considerations, but the request for reduced laboratory charges met with 'a curt refusal'.[18] Saunders conceded that 'our efforts to control the disease has been greatly limited by this factor [...] we are therefore thrown back upon the only logical remedy which is the mass immunization of the whole community'.[19]

Despite the best efforts of the Cork public health department, the most enduring obstacle to attaining communal protection against diphtheria lay with the widespread reluctance of parents to present their children for immunization treatment. Saunders commented:

What is to be said about this? Is it ignorance or lethargy or the result of the propaganda of misguided zealots? Whatever the source the effect is deplorable. It seems impossible to bring home to the majority of people their responsibilities in such matters and still we have had ample personal experience of the remorse of parents whose children have died from diphtheria. If any means could be devised to bring the feelings of such parents to the notice of indifferent individuals the efforts of propagandists would not survive long. It is an unfortunate fact that, only when confronted with the actual danger, can most parents be roused from their indifference.[20]

The 1942 outbreak certainly roused parents from their 'indifference'. The disease made its appearance in epidemic form and the accompanying fatalities caused parents to become alive to what was happening in a way that no

17 Saunders, *Report 1942*, 18.
18 *Irish Times*, 11 June 1942.
19 Saunders, *Report 1942*, 20–21.
20 Saunders, *Report 1942*, 16.

previous warning was able to effect. During 1942, 6,871 children presented for treatment. This necessitated over 15,000 individual attendances at the public health clinic, placing a strain on staff and disrupting routine work. Over the course of the year, 4,000 children completed a full course of treatment; the remainder being previously treated children returning for re-test, or further treatment where necessary.[21] Despite record attendances, the epidemic continued unabated into 1943 and incidence remained high throughout the year. A further 326 cases occurred during 1943 and 17 fatalities ensued. Again, not a single victim was an immunized child.[22] The concentration of immunization treatment on children of school-going age again effected increased incidence among adolescents and adults. While this age group accounted for 15 per cent of all cases in 1942, this increased substantially to 46 per cent of all cases in 1943. The corresponding decrease in the rate of incidence among children of school-going age, from 57 per cent in 1942 to 39.5 per cent in 1943, indicates that immunization work undertaken in the city schools succeeded in stemming incidence among schoolchildren.[23] This reduction would become more apparent in subsequent years.

The acute emergency during 1942 motivated large numbers of parents to present children for immunization treatment. Although the epidemic continued into 1943, the numbers presented for treatment that year decreased to 1,387. This downward trend continued during 1944, when just 734 children received full immunization treatment. The epidemic began to wane in the closing weeks of 1943, and continued to diminish during 1944, when 172 cases and five fatalities occurred. The resultant case fatality rate of 2.9 per cent was one of the lowest diphtheria mortality rates recorded in the city in the preceding fifty-five years. Saunders opined that the strain of diphtheria prevalent in the city had become less virulent, or, that the child population of the city had greatly increased their immunity to the disease. Analysis of incidence during 1944 supports the latter explanation.

Over the three years 1942–44, a diminished incidence of diphtheria occurred among schoolchildren, falling from 57 per cent of all cases in 1942, to 39.5 per cent in 1943, and to 27 per cent in 1944. For the first time in the recorded history of the city, no diphtheria fatality occurred in the four-eight-year-old age group during the year, the age group that traditionally sustained the greatest amount of fatalities. Conversely, incidence among adolescents and adults continued to rise. Over the corresponding period, incidence among these groupings increased from 15 per cent of all cases in 1942, to

21 Saunders, *Report 1942*, 20–21.
22 CCCLS/352.4. J. C. Saunders, *Report of the Medical Officer of Health for the year 1943*, 12.
23 Saunders, *Report 1943*, 17.

46 per cent in 1943, and accounted for almost 63 per cent of cases during 1944. In this sense, diphtheria had followed the same pattern as smallpox; immunization altered the characteristics of the disease.

In 1945, a substantial decrease in diphtheria morbidity and mortality occurred. Ninety-six cases notified and five deaths ensued. A further and more dramatic reduction occurred in 1946, with 46 reported cases and two fatalities.[24] Although Saunders thought these figures 'satisfactory', he regarded the two fatalities as 'unnecessary deaths', and the diminution in the numbers of children presenting for treatment continued to cause him some concern.[25] Notwithstanding this, the downward trend in diphtheria morbidity and mortality continued during 1947. Eighteen cases occurred during the year, setting a new low record for diphtheria in the city. More importantly, for the first time in the statistical history of the city, no diphtheria mortality occurred. Saunders hailed this result 'the second last landmark towards the ultimate objective – the complete elimination of the disease'.[26]

Trends that defined the relationship between the rate of diphtheria morbidity and the rate of anti-diphtheria immunization made Saunders uneasy. Although satisfied with the 'present happy position' Saunders was apprehensive that low levels of incidence would induce low levels of attendance at the immunization clinic, and that 'it is only a question of time as to when the disease will again assume serious proportions'.[27] Saunders's fears were unfounded. The historically low morbidity and mortality rates continued their downward trend, and importantly, attendances at the immunization clinic held steady. As a result, the city remained free from diphtheria mortality for the five years 1947–51. The correlation between anti-diphtheria immunization and the complete absence of diphtheria related fatalities was not lost on parents, and annual attendances at the municipal immunization clinic almost doubled from 787 to 1,442 over the corresponding period.[28]

Five diphtheria cases occurred in the city during 1952 and despite the record low incidence two fatalities ensued.[29] One victim was eight months

24 CCCLS/352.4. J. C. Saunders, *Report of the Medical Officer of Health for the year 1946*, 12.

25 Saunders, *Report 1946*, 12. Both fatalities recorded during 1946 occurred in children aged between two and four years.

26 CCCLS/352.4. J. C. Saunders, *Report of the Medical Officer of Health for the year 1947*, Section VI, Infectious disease.

27 WLAM/b.13556794. J. C. Saunders, *Report of the Medical Officer of Health for the year 1948*, 26.

28 CCCLS/352.4. J. C. Saunders, *Report of the Medical Officer of Health for the year 1951*, 27.

29 CCCLS/352.4. J. C. Saunders, *Report of the Medical Officer of Health for the year 1952*, 23.

old, and the other was a child of three years. The infant was the youngest of three children, and the only non-immunized child in the family. In both cases, the disease had an 'insidious onset' and advanced too far for treatment before parents summoned medical aid. That diphtheria could infiltrate a family and pick out the only unimmunized child served to highlight the treacherous nature of the disease, and these two fatalities, which interrupted a sequence of five consecutive years without a diphtheria fatality, served to create increased parental demand for immunization treatment. In response, a special effort by the school medical officer, Dr Curtain, and his staff met with a considerable degree of success and the number of children presenting for preventive treatment during the year more than doubled.[30]

In 1953, just one diphtheria case occurred and there were no case fatalities in the city.[31] Although numbers presenting for immunization treatment reduced because of a more urgent BCG campaign in the city schools, in general, an average of 1,366 children continued to present for anti-diphtheria immunization treatment annually.[32] Considering the average annual live birth rate in the city was 1,509 during the early 1950s it is possible to deduce that 90.5 per cent of the city's new-borns presented annually for anti-diphtheria immunization treatment. Herd immunity ensued and incidence fell to negligible numbers. Immunization consigned diphtheria to memory in this city.

> Taking into consideration the epidemic waves of the disease which scourged the city in former years this may be regarded as a notable achievement. How long this happy state of affairs is liable to remain it is impossible to say. It will depend largely on the co-operation of parents in our diphtheria immunization scheme. Our present position is entirely attributable to this scheme. We know that the diphtheria bacillus has not been eliminated, sporadic cases of the disease afford us the warning, whether it will ever assume epidemic form will depend entirely on the number of children who are immunised.[33]
>
> John Charles Saunders, 1953.

30 Saunders, *Report 1952*, 24.
31 CCCLS/352.4. J. C. Saunders, *Report of the Medical Officer of Health for the year 1953*, 22.
32 CCCLS/352.4. J. C. Saunders, *Report of the Medical Officer of Health for the year 1954*, 30.
33 Saunders, *Report 1953*, 2–3.

Dublin

The Ring tragedy exacted a heavy toll on all established immunization schemes in Ireland, but affected Dublin most acutely. Anti-diphtheria immunization was freely available in the city since 1930, and by the end of 1937, 63,416 children received treatment. The 1936 census estimates that Dublin city's child population comprised 50,645 children and infants aged four years or younger; 42,338 children aged five to nine years and 42,622 aged 10–14 years. In a city that registered around 11,600 live births per year, contemporary immunization rates did not make for a hopeful augury.[34] The dramatic falloff in the number of children presented for treatment, combined with the withdrawal of immunization services by the Irish Medical Union, resulted in much increased diphtheria morbidity and mortality in Dublin. During 1938, 958 cases occurred and 92 fatalities ensued. These figures elicited an admission from the municipal medical officer, Matt Russell, that 'no real improvement was possible' even though anti-immunization schemes were available in the city for the previous nine years. Russell again blamed the failure of the schemes on parents who did not avail of facilities provided by the public health clinics for the protection of infants and young children.[35] Despite undertaking a citywide propaganda campaign in 1938, numbers attending the immunization clinics fell even further, with little over 3,800 attendances recorded.

Diminishing immunization rates, and the endemic and virulent nature of diphtheria in Dublin, combined to create a highly volatile situation. During 1938, fewer than 2.5 per cent of the city's general child population, and little more than 0.5 per cent of the total population of the city received immunizing treatment.[36] The number of immunized children represented little more than a fraction of the actual number of children living in the city, children who endured a prolonged and virulent diphtheria epidemic. It is probable that a high proportion of diphtheria carriers permeated the school-going population, creating a deadly environment for children entering school life. It is unsurprising then that the majority of diphtheria cases recorded during 1939 and 1940 occurred among schoolchildren. Notwithstanding this, pre-school children and infants continued to bear the brunt of the disease, accounting for over 50 per cent of case fatalities reported during both years.[37]

34 Russell, *Dublin Report 1937*, 42.
35 Matthew J. Russell, *Report on the state of public health in the City of Dublin for the year 1938* (Dublin, 1939), 12.
36 Russell, *Dublin Report 1938*, 12.
37 Matthew J. Russell, *Report on the state of public health in the City of Dublin for the two years ending 31ˢᵗ December 1940* (Dublin, 1941), 39–41.

During 1939, Russell pleaded with Dublin dispensary doctors to use their 'favourable position' in their relations with mothers and guardians of young children, so that their 'undoubted influence' might induce them to present children for immunization treatment. Russell 'sincerely hoped' that private practitioners would find themselves in a position to give their 'complete and enthusiastic cooperation in this very important work'. However, as dispensary doctors were still embroiled in a bitter dispute with the DLG&PH regarding immunization fees, cooperation, enthusiastic or otherwise, was not forthcoming from that particular section of the medical community.[38] Even if Russell secured their cooperation, it was widely accepted that the dispensary system in Dublin was 'extraordinarily inefficient'.[39] Every year, thousands of patients, warranting medical attention at city dispensaries, had no option but to present at outpatients' departments in the city's voluntary hospitals, where acutely sick patients routinely mixed openly with those with minor complaints. This not only created increased opportunities for the propagation of infectious disease, but it placed extreme pressure on hospital services. Acutely ill and sometimes dying children were turned away daily from the doors of children's hospitals, 'to be carried back to tenement rooms, because beds were already filled'.[40]

These insurmountable factors forced Russell to fall back on resources under his own control. A more energetic propaganda campaign promoting the benefits of anti-diphtheria immunization during 1939 secured the cooperation of 6,177 parents. Although this was an increase of over 100 per cent on the previous year, it represented only a fraction of the 30,934 attendances secured during 1935. Although attendances remained steady during 1940, diphtheria remained epidemic throughout the city.[41] During 1941, over 440 diphtheria cases presented at Cork Street Fever Hospital alone: 39 proved fatal. The superintendent at Cork Street, Christopher McSweeney reported:

For those who see several fresh cases of diphtheria every day, many of them desperately ill with the severer forms of the disease, it is disheartening in the extreme to realise the indifference which parents display towards the only effective method of coping with this preventable disease [...] The authorities have provided the facilities. It is for the parents to use them. The death of a child from diphtheria

38 Russell, *Dublin Report 1939/1940*, 6.
39 W. R. F. Collis, 'Some facts and figures in relation to health in Dublin', *Irish Journal of Medical Science*, No. 173 (May 1940), 193–200.
40 Collis, *Irish Journal of Medical Science* (1940), 198.
41 Russell, *Dublin Report 1939/1940*, 41.

nowadays carries with it some implication of neglect on the parts of the parents.[42]

In May 1941, aerial bombardment of Dublin by the Luftwaffe caused mass destruction of property and necessitated the re-location of 1,712 people. Many found accommodation in the Red Cross Refuge, most moved in with friends and family, but in all cases, this meant the transfer of children to new schools and new surroundings.[43] Fear that further bombing raids would ensue, and the realization that an emergency evacuation of children from the city was an increasingly real prospect, caused alarm among public health officials. The Dublin health department prepared to deal with such an eventuality with the proviso that prospective evacuees submit for full anti-diphtheria immunization treatment.[44] Diphtheria posed a far greater threat to the child population of Dublin than anything the Luftwaffe could throw at them, and between 5 May and 20 June 1941 47,000 children received treatment in the form of two injections of APT. By the end of the year, a record 50,027 presented for treatment.[45]

During this period of acute emergency, the prospect of further air attacks, and possible military invasion, prompted the Civil Defence Authorities to seriously consider the evacuation of 120,000 children from Dublin city, and to disperse them among the rural population. While potential urban evacuees would have developed high levels of acquired immunity against diphtheria, and received additional protection through immunization, it is highly probable that a significant proportion were carriers of virulent diphtheria bacilli. Unlike their British counterparts, the Irish Civil Defence Authorities made no provision to immunize children in the prospective, and predominantly rural, host communities. Fortunately, civil evacuation was unnecessary, and in all probability, averted a major public health disaster.[46]

The prophylactic utilized in the 1941 campaign was Burroughs Wellcome APT antigen, administered in two doses, and a major feature of the campaign was that more than 50 per cent of children failed to return for their second shot. Analysis of the wartime anti-diphtheria campaign in Dublin for the years 1941–44 reveals that 212,427 children presented for immunization

42 Winslow Sterling-Berry, 'Reports of medical inspectors on the public health of the districts under their charge', DLG&PH, *Report 1941–42*, 167.
43 Catherine O'Brien, *Annual report of the school medical service for the year ended 31st December 1944* (County Borough of Dublin, 1945), 3.
44 Matthew J. Russell, *Report on the state of public health in the City of Dublin for the year 1944* (Dublin, 1945), 40.
45 James C. Gaffney, 'A statistical study of the epidemiology and prevention of diphtheria in Dublin; Part I', *Irish Journal of Medical Science*, No. 208 (April 1943), 97–115.
46 Gaffney, *Irish Journal of Medical Science* (April 1943), 98.

treatment, but just 98,821, or a little over 46 per cent, received the full course. The wartime intervention during the latter half of 1941 certainly made a positive impact in lessening the incidence of diphtheria in the city – in fact incidence was reduced by almost 50 per cent – but, as the threat of further bombings lessened, so too did the number of children attending municipal immunization clinics.

A further complication during this period was that the percentage of immunized children who subsequently contracted diphtheria began to rise. Between 1941 and 1944, incidence of post-treatment diphtheria rose from 12.3 per cent per annum to 18.7 per cent per annum suggesting that immunization with Wellcome's APT antigen failed to protect one in every five treated children. While a report compiled by one medical officer, A. F. Cooney, stated that the increase could be put down to, 'increased virulence in these years' it is likely that the substantial non-completion rate instilled a false sense of security among parents.[47] As a result, during 1943 and 1944, diphtheria returned in epidemic proportions, registering the highest incidence ever recorded in the city.

In January 1943, Matt Russell met with Dublin City Council to discuss the increasing incidence of diphtheria in the city.[48] Here, a number of practical, administrative, and promotional suggestions were agreed. Firstly, anti-diphtheria immunization facilities extended to include additional weekly one-hour sessions at six different centres, a bi-weekly one-hour session at one centre and a tri-weekly session at the Child Welfare Centre on Lord Edward Street.[49] The health department sanctioned the employment of additional part-time medical officers, nurses, and clerks to treat schoolchildren continually during school term. In addition, the public health department would send a letter to the mother or guardian of every child on its first birthday outlining the reasons why the child should be immunized, including a list of the centres where immunization was available free of charge.[50] Russell instituted an advertising campaign in the press, on hoardings, and in public transport vehicles operating in the city, outlining the facilities available for immunization. Corporation health visitors agreed to use their position to urge mothers to present children at immunization centres for treatment, and medical officers, and nurses engaged at Maternity and Child Welfare Clinics, undertook to advise and encourage mothers to have children immunized.[51]

47 Russell, *Dublin Report 1944*, 41.
48 NAI, B 34/63 Vol. I, Notes on a conference regarding the incidence of diphtheria in Dublin County Borough, 28 January 1943.
49 Lord Edward Street is now Dame Street.
50 Notes on a conference regarding the incidence of diphtheria in Dublin County Borough.
51 Russell, *Dublin Report 1944*, 38–39.

These efforts combined secured 41,138 attendances during 1943; however, little more than 45 per cent completed a full course of treatment. Relatively low attendance rates, high rates of partial immunization treatment, and general wartime conditions conspired against Russell and his department, and an unprecedented 1,345 diphtheria cases notified in 1943, an increase of 100 per cent on the previous year and the highest incidence on record for the city. The DLG&PH regarded the deteriorating position in relation to the prevalence of diphtheria in Dublin as a 'very grave' situation. Minister, Séan MacEntee, cautioned Dublin City Manager, Patrick Hernon, that all municipal medical staff were expected to make every effort to combat diphtheria, and insisted on the application of all available machinery for propaganda and treatment 'to arrest the spreading havoc that it was causing in the city of Dublin'.[52] Russell urged the minister to settle the long running dispute with the Irish Medical Association (formerly the Irish Medical Union) which would allow dispensary medical officers, and general practitioners, to administer anti-diphtheria antitoxin with remuneration from the department. MacEntee dismissed Russell's proposal on the grounds that 'it did not appear to be feasible'.[53]

Eschewing Russell's call for increased assistance from private medical practitioners, MacEntee instead mooted the much more frugal possibility of ecclesiastical assistance, dispatching a correspondence to Archbishop John Charles McQuaid seeking his support in utilizing parish priests to extol the benefits of active immunization to their parishioners. When no reply was forthcoming, MacEntee sent a representative, Dr Morgan Crowe, to meet with the archbishop to impress on him the seriousness of the situation in relation to diphtheria in the city. While Crowe received a sympathetic hearing, the archbishop somewhat providentially replied that 'the worst of the epidemic had passed' and refrained from making any commitment to assist. MacEntee was convinced that the clergy had an important role to play, and indeed a civic duty to promote anti-diphtheria services in the city, and concluded that the only possible explanation was that Dr Crowe had not sufficiently conveyed the seriousness of the situation to the archbishop. However, a subsequent meeting between MacEntee and McQuaid came to a similarly unfruitful conclusion, and the prospect of ecclesiastic aid was quietly shelved.[54]

The extended immunization services rolled out during 1943 succeeded in facilitating increased numbers presenting for treatment during 1944.

52 NAI, B 34/63 Vol. I, Note by DLG&PH Inspector Winslow Sterling-Berry.
53 NAI, B 34/63 Vol. I, Notes on a conference regarding the incidence of diphtheria in Dublin County Borough.
54 NAI, B 34/63 Vol. I. Minutes of the Public Health Department of Dublin County Borough, and notes written by Winslow Sterling-Berry, and John MacCormack DLG&PH.

Almost 60,000 children presented for treatment during the year, however, the non-completion rate remained high, as did the rate of incidence, which stood at 1,326 cases. For the years 1943–44, 155 children lost their lives to diphtheria in Dublin: 147 received no immunization treatment.[55] The extraordinary increase in diphtheria notifications during these years placed enormous pressure on the city fever hospitals, which recorded their highest number of admissions on record. Cork Street Fever Hospital turned away 689 cases of infectious disease because of lack of accommodation. Of the 2,613 patients who gained admittance, 250 fatalities ensued, and 44 were diphtheria related. To curtail the spread of diphtheria, hospital administrators barred parental visits for the duration of a child's illness and parents followed their child's progress through reports in the evening newspapers.[56] Christopher McSweeney stated that diphtheria fatalities in Cork Street Fever Hospital were 'a disgrace to any enlightened community-implying a degree of apathy, amounting to neglect', and called on the DLG&PH to introduce compulsory immunization and booster-immunizations during the first ten years of child life.[57] Fine Gael TD, Maurice Dockrell, raised McSweeney's proposal in Dáil Éireann. Parliamentary secretary to the DLG&PH, Dr Con Ward, replied that he could not make any statement concerning compulsory immunization treatment; however, he asserted that 'the present arrangements for immunization were receiving close investigation in his department'.[58]

At Vergemount Fever Hospital, Clonskeagh, resident medical superintendent, F. N. Elcock, reported that diphtheria patients accounted for 36 per cent of all admissions, and 46 per cent of hospital mortalities, during 1944. Of 1,591 admissions to Vergemount during the year, 569 were diphtheria cases, 37 of which proved fatal. St Gerard's Home on Herbert Avenue was opened during 1942 to house convalescent diphtheria patients, and the increasing and sustained pressure exerted on hospital facilities necessitated the opening of an old play-hall with the intention of accommodating 12 children. By 1944, the converted hall contained 36 fully occupied beds, and although far from being an ideal situation, this facility freed up beds at Vergemount to treat ever-growing numbers of acute diphtheria cases.[59]

Close to 50 per cent of Vergemount's diphtheria fatalities occurred in children deemed 'beyond medical aid' on admission. In the majority of these cases, children presented for admission to hospital on or after the third day of illness, and many more on the fifth day or later. Some cases, haemorrhagic

55 Russell, *Dublin Report 1944*, 41–42.
56 Farmar, *Patients, potions and physicians*, 159.
57 'Diphtheria death "a disgrace"', *Irish Times*, 1 July 1944.
58 'Post-War building industry', *Irish Times*, 19 October 1944.
59 F.N. Elcock, *Vergemount Fever Hospital Clonskeagh, Annual report for the year ended, 31 December 1944*, in Russell, *Dublin Report 1944*, 45.

in origin, did not respond to treatment, while the remaining cases were of a toxic or laryngeal type of diphtheria, and presented too late to benefit from treatment.[60] Previous experience with the disease at Vergemount had shown that the chances of recovering from a toxic case of diphtheria were slim after three days had passed before the administration of antitoxin. Of the 37 diphtheria related fatalities admitted to Vergemount during 1944, 36 had not availed of anti-diphtheria immunization treatment. Vergemount introduced diphtheria treatment combining active and passive immunity during 1940. However, war conditions made it difficult to procure supplies of the anti-diphtheria antigen Formol Toxoid, forcing Vergemount to abandon active immunization. The administration of antitoxin to children in the first days of illness proved successful, reducing fatalities and influencing a reduction in the frequency of paralyses. Early admission to hospital spared the lives of many children who had not previously received anti-diphtheria immunization treatment. However, diphtheria often left its mark in the form of paralyses, fatal forms of broncho-pneumonia, and permanently weakened hearts.[61]

Analysis of the 37 diphtheria fatalities recorded at Vergemount during 1944 reveals that all occurred in children and infants aged between thirteen days and nine years: all but six children were aged five years or younger. In no case was a fatal case admitted to Vergemount before the third day of illness, and in one instance, sixteen days had passed before parents presented the child. In every case, the hospital reports make for grim reading. In two instances, infants aged 13 and 15 days presented with diphtheria complicated by enteritis and diarrhoea. Both died some days after admission. A nine-month old infant admitted on the third day of illness with nasal diphtheria, complicated by broncho-pneumonia, died on admission. A nine-month old infant admitted on the fifth day of illness, 'ashen grey in colour' and in an extremely toxic state, died within twenty-four hours of admission. An eleven-month old infant admitted on the sixth day of illness was reportedly 'moribund on admission', suffering from laryngeal and nasal diphtheria. A tracheotomy was performed which gave some relief, but death from cardiac failure ensued within 24 hours. A five-year-old admitted on the third day of illness with faucal and nasal diphtheria collapsed and died from acute cardiac failure.[62]

Among the diphtheria related fatalities recorded at Vergemount, no child received preventive anti-diphtheria immunization treatment. Preventive

60 Elcock, *Vergemount Report 1944*, 47.
61 Elcock, *Vergemount Report 1944*, 48. See also, Stuyvesant Butler and Samuel A. Levine, 'Diphtheria as a cause of late heart-block', *American Heart Journal*, Vol. 5, No. 5 (June 1930), 592–698.
62 Elcock, *Vergemount Report 1944*, 48.

treatment with antitoxin had proved successful in absorbing circulating diphtheria toxin, and toxin loosely combined with tissue. However, the administration of antitoxin in an already stricken child proved less effective in absorbing toxin firmly combined with tissue. The length of postponement in seeking medical treatment had a direct and relative impact on the efficacy, or otherwise, of anti-diphtheria prophylactic. Every fatal diphtheria case admitted to Vergemount during 1944 was associated with a delayed hospital admission. All presented in an extremely toxic state, gasping for breath owing to a marked obstruction in the throat, and in every case death resulted from acute cardiac failure.[63]

In April 1944, a consignment of medical supplies sent by the American Red Cross reached the Irish Red Cross Society in Dublin. This, the seventh consignment received since the outbreak of the war, included a wide assortment of surgical instruments, 15 operating tables, 4.5 tons of insulin, 500,000 vitamin tablets, 2,500,000 sulphanilamide tablets, and 45,500,000 diphtheria serum units.[64] The Red Cross consignment eased any fears relating to the supply of anti-diphtheria antigens and facilitated a further intensification of anti-diphtheria immunization services in Dublin. For the three years to April 1947, services extended to include 11 weekly immunization sessions at eight different locations, which in the main catered for children aged under two years. To complement the work of the immunization clinics, medical officers made regular visits to 86 city schools, averaging 180 visits annually. Health visitors continued to advocate immunization to parents. Notices and explanatory propaganda appeared in the daily press every few months, and almost 13,000 infants received 'birthday cards' to remind parents of the municipal immunization services available to them. Additional measures introduced to stem the propagation of the disease involved the identification of diphtheria contacts, who were then suspended from school for a week, and the identification of diphtheria contacts working with food, who were excluded from their duties pending the result of bacterial throat swab analysis.[65] On his retirement from an extended stint as chief medical officer in April 1947, Matt Russell could take some satisfaction from the fact that the sustained and concerted effort to exercise a level of control over diphtheria in Dublin had met with some, albeit belated, success. For the years 1944–47, incidence steadily declined, falling from 1,330 cases in 1944, to 185 cases in 1947.[66] Although 50 of the 185 confirmed cases gave a history

63 Elcock, *Vergemount Report 1944*, 49–52.
64 'Red Cross supplies from America', *Irish Times*, 3 April 1944.
65 Morgan P. Crowe (Acting MOH), *Report on the state of public health in the City of Dublin for the year 1947* (Dublin, 1949), 28.
66 Crowe, *Dublin Report 1947*, 22.

of previous immunization, Russell considered the improvement as 'one of the brightest features of our communicable disease control efforts'.

In June 1947, the newly established Department of Health issued a circular to every county and municipal medical officer in the state mandating the implementation of anti-diphtheria immunization programmes in their districts if they had not already done so. The circular advised on how to undertake a safe and effective immunization scheme, but notably it also included a provision whereby medical officers could provide antitoxin and active immunization material free of charge to all medical practitioners in their districts.[67] Dublin Corporation immediately made immunizing agents available to general practitioners for the treatment of suspected diphtheria cases, and for the protection of known contacts. While the number of children treated by private practitioners during the latter part of 1947 is indeterminable, the public health department conceded that numbers were 'undoubtedly quite considerable'.[68]

In a further development, in February 1948, a coalition government, consisting of Fine Gael, the Labour Party, Clann na Talmhan, Clann na Poblachta, National Labour, and independents broke Fianna Fail's sixteen-year monopoly on Irish politics. Among the many first-time TD's elected, a 32-year-old doctor, Noel Browne, became Minister of the newly established Department of Health. In office, Browne sought to highlight 'the inertia of both Fianna Fáil and Fine Gael in providing a service for preventable diseases'.[69] He was determined to transform the department into 'a battle headquarters' and is remembered for his central role in the crusade against tuberculosis in Ireland, and the ill-fated, for Browne at least, Mother and Child Scheme.[70] An early and little known, political intervention by Browne succeeded in brokering a deal with the Irish Medical Association, ending the twelve-year dispute with central health regarding immunization fees. Browne's recommendation that a substantial increase in fees be paid to general practitioners for their anti-diphtheria immunization work acquiesced to the medical professions resistance to what J. J. Lee termed 'cheap medicine',[71] a point which Browne seems to have overlooked during the Mother and Child controversy two years later.[72]

For the 12 years to 1948, general practitioners carried out immunization schemes only where a local medical officer declared that a state

---

67 NAI, B 34/63 Vol. I, Circular P.H. 17/47.
68 Crowe, *Dublin Report 1947*, 28.
69 Noel Browne, *Against the tide* (Dublin, 1986), 99.
70 For analysis of Noel Browne and the Mother and Child controversy, see John Horgan, *Noel Browne: Passionate outsider* (Dublin, 2000).
71 J. J. Lee, *Ireland 1912–1985: Politics and society* (Cambridge, 1989), 315.
72 'How Dublin will benefit from new health plan', *Irish Times*, 1 May 1948.

of emergency was present due to the existence of diphtheria in epidemic form.[73] As medical officers were slow to declare that a 'state of emergency' existed in their district, general practitioners did not receive many requests of this nature. Following Browne's intervention in May 1948, the executive committee of the medical association issued a statement to their members that read: 'Due to the co-operation and understanding of the Minister for Health and the Department officials in the Ministry [...] we advise doctors to carry out now a routine scheme of immunization willingly and speedily'.[74] The Department of Health made supplies of anti-diphtheritic serum freely available to medical practitioners throughout the state to treat suspected cases of diphtheria and the victim's immediate contacts. The vast majority of diphtheria related fatalities occurred in children presenting for medical attention at an advanced stage of disease. The cooperation of general practitioners, now armed with supplies of anti-diphtheria serum, meant that afflicted children received antitoxin treatment as soon as they presented at a dispensary, thereby substantially increasing their chances of survival. In addition, immediately identifying, and immunizing close contacts curtailed scope for the further propagation of the disease.

In Dublin, the positive results attendant on Browne's intervention were immediate. During 1948, fewer than 100 diphtheria cases occurred and just one diphtheria related fatality ensued. Despite a record number of hospital admissions that year, few were diphtheria cases.[75] Vergemount admitted 2,245 patients during 1948, only eight of which were diphtheria cases.[76] This represented 0.35 per cent of total admissions to Vergemount for the year, a remarkable reduction on figures recorded just four years earlier when diphtheria cases represented 36 per cent of admissions to the same institution. In 1949, Vergemount admitted no diphtheria case, and an even more notable achievement was that, for the first time in the history of the city, Dublin city recorded no diphtheria related mortality.[77]

For the six years to 1954, diphtheria is largely absent from Dublin's statistical record, and apart from one fatality in an unimmunized child during 1950, the city remained free of diphtheria mortality. During the corresponding period, scarlet fever, measles, and whooping cough appeared in epidemic form throughout the city. While these diseases historically

73 'Doctors accept Department's terms', *Irish Times*, 3 May 1948.
74 *Irish Times*, 3 May 1948.
75 James A. Harbison, *Report of the Medical Officer of Health, City of Dublin, for the year 1948* (Dublin, 1950), 12.
76 F. N. Elcock, *Vergemount Fever Hospital, Annual report for the year ended 31 December 1948*, in Harbison, *Report 1948*, 53.
77 James A. Harbison, *Report of the City Medical Officer, City of Dublin, for the year 1951* (Dublin, 1952), 6.

appeared in cyclical waves, by 1954, they appeared annually and almost 37,000 children were hospitalized with one, or other, of these afflictions over this six-year period.[78] This sustained attack relegated diphtheria, and by extension anti-diphtheria immunization, to a less prominent place in the public consciousness, and because diphtheria reduced substantially, there was an accompanying public perception that anti-diphtheria immunization treatment was no longer a necessity.[79]

As a result, in the spring of 1954, a short, sharp outbreak of the more serious gravis form of diphtheria occurred among a group of unimmunized children in Dublin. Seventeen cases occurred and three fatalities ensued.[80] Despite renewed press and radio propaganda designed to impress on parents that it was incumbent upon them to have their children protected against diphtheria, the warnings went largely unheeded. Diphtheria reappeared late in 1954 and continued into 1955 claiming two more lives.[81] In response, the public health department promoted combined immunization against whooping cough and diphtheria, a move that induced many parents to present children for immunization treatment due to the prevalence of whooping cough in the city in the preceding years.[82]

End of an Epidemic

In 1947, the newly established Department of Health ushered in several important changes in health administration under the Health Act 1947. The provision of public health legislation relating to housing, water supply, sewage, and other sanitary services remained under the auspices of the Department of Local Government. However, matters relating to the provision of medical services for mothers and children, the prevention of infectious disease, the provision of institutions by health authorities, and the appointment of county medical officers came under the remit of the Department of Health.[83] In relation to infectious disease and infestation, part IV of the Health Act empowered the Minister to define infectious diseases and to make regulations to prevent their

78 James A. Harbison, *Report of the City Medical Officer, City of Dublin, for the year 1954* (Dublin, 1955), 6.
79 Harbison, *Report 1954*, 10.
80 'Virulent type of diphtheria', *Irish Times*, 10 March 1954.
81 'Diphtheria still a menace', *Irish Times*, 23 November 1954. 'Diphtheria danger not past', *Irish Times*, 29 November 1954.
82 Harbison, *Report 1954*, 10. 'Parents now see the danger', *Irish Times*, 16 March 1954. 'Diphtheria reports rouse parents', *Irish Times*, 31 March 1954. '57 cases of whooping cough', *Irish Times*, 22 December 1955.
83 Department of Health, *First Report 1945–1949* (Dublin, 1951), 33–34.

spread. These provisions provided a basis for the introduction or expansion of schemes designed to tackle diseases such as diphtheria, typhoid, measles, tuberculosis, and venereal disease. While the new legislation contained a provision to exempt conscientious objectors from participating in immunization schemes, it also contained a proviso that in exceptional circumstances, all persons could be compelled to undergo immunization treatment to ensure that outbreaks of disease were contained locally, and eradicated.[84]

On 1 April 1948, the Infectious Disease Regulations introduced legislation designed to protect against diphtheria, smallpox, and other diseases by means of immunization and vaccination. These measures directed health authorities to supply approved diagnostic and immunizing agents to persons living in their districts, to medical officers of health, and to private practitioners. In addition, Article 24 of the regulations empowered chief medical officers to immunize all children against diphtheria, without right of exemption, should they decide that the severity of an outbreak warranted such intervention. These measures indicated that the incumbent interparty coalition government was inclined to take a stringent, and if necessary, interventionist approach to the control of infectious disease in general, and to diphtheria in particular.[85]

Health minister Noel Browne maintained that active immunization was the best method available to exert a degree of control over diphtheria, although he equally acknowledged that arrangements for anti-diphtheria immunization services in the state were 'spasmodic and rather haphazard'. In response, a more regular and systematic national anti-diphtheria immunization programme was organized on the principal feature that immunization was, and would remain, a free public health service. The department determined that the choice of prophylactic used should be at the sole discretion of the chief medical officer in each district and that propaganda by advertisement and personal approach to families was an essential element of the campaign. Health departments were to offer immunization services at local dispensaries, schools, and other centres selected by the chief medical officer, who would stress the importance of early immunization and urge parents to give infants their first immunization course at between nine and twelve months old. In addition, the department directed that any doctor could obtain antitoxin and active immunization material free of charge on condition that they supply returns of all immunizations, complete with details of the material supplied, to the health authority.[86]

84 Department of Health, *First Report*, 34.
85 The previous Fianna Fáil administration introduced these measures in the *Health Bill, 1945*. The *Health Act 1947* brought the provisions of the bill into law.
86 Department of Health, 'The infectious disease service', *First Report*, 47.

The minister urged all local health authorities to operate these arrangements 'intensively' and dispatched department medical inspectors to monitor progress in various counties and to intervene to solve any local difficulties encountered. This concerted effort produced favourable results. The number of children presented for immunization treatment in the state almost doubled from 42,000 in 1946 to 80,000 in 1948,[87] and a persistent downward trend in national diphtheria rates ensued: falling from 521 cases and 30 deaths in 1948 to 28 cases and seven deaths in 1952.[88]

Reports in the medical and daily press, alleging a connection between anti-diphtheria immunization and poliomyelitis elicited a brief, albeit 'disturbing effect' on the national scheme during 1950. During the year, separate investigations undertaken by Geffen,[89] Martin,[90] and McCloskey[91] suggested a possible connection between intramuscular injections and a flaccid paralysis of one limb, as experienced by polio victims.[92] A subsequent statistical investigation undertaken by Bradford Hill and Knowelden in England and Wales found there was 'clearly an association between recent injections and paralysis', influencing the British Ministry of Health to halt anti-diphtheria immunization in districts where poliomyelitis was prevalent.[93] British newspapers were unambiguous in their assertion that diphtheria immunization 'caused poliomyelitis' and according to some commentators 'the reaction amongst mothers was immediate'.[94] A contributor to the *British Medical Journal* observed 'Those who are intelligent were naturally anxious but still wished to have their babies immunized against diphtheria after being assured. The others (and those, alas with the largest families) of lower intelligence [...] have immediately clutched at this excuse and nothing will ever make them agree to immunization now'.[95]

87 Department of Health, *First Report*, 48.
88 Department of Health, *Health progress 1947–1953* (Dublin, 1953), 17.
89 D. H. Geffen, 'The incidence of paralysis occurring in London children within four weeks after immunization', *Medical Officer*, Vol. 83 (8 April 1950), 137–40.
90 J. K. Martin, 'Local paralysis in children after injections', *Archives of Disease in Childhood*, Vol. 25, No. 121 (1950), 1–14.
91 Bertram P. McCloskey, 'The relation of prophylactic inoculations to the onset of poliomyelitis', *The Lancet*, Vol. 255, No. 6606 (8 April 1950), 659–63.
92 'Poliomyelitis after immunization', *British Medical Journal* (15 April 1950), 890–91.
93 A. Bradford Hill and J. Knowelden, 'Inoculation and poliomyelitis: A statistical investigation in England and Wales in 1949', *British Medical Journal* (1 July 1950), 1–6. See also, H. Stanley Banks and A. J. Beale, 'Poliomyelitis and immunization against whooping cough and diphtheria', *BMJ* (29 July 1950), 251–52; Marguerite Darnton, 'Immunization and poliomyelitis', *BMJ* (24 June 1950), 1489; and Robert Cruickshank, 'Poliomyelitis after immunization', *BMJ* (13 May 1950), 1139.
94 Mary E. Budding, 'Immunization and poliomyelitis', *British Medical Journal* (27 May 1950), 1273.
95 Budding, *British Medical Journal* (1950), 1273.

In Belfast, a retrospective investigation of a previous poliomyelitis epidemic, undertaken by the senior medical officer for the city, W. J. McLeod, failed to establish any association between immunization and paralysis, and health authorities there continued with their anti-diphtheria immunization despite the presence of poliomyelitis in epidemic form.[96] In Dublin, the Department of Health requested chief medical officers to submit particulars of every case of poliomyelitis to come to their attention in previous years, and following an examination of previous polio outbreaks, the department arrived at similar conclusions as their Belfast counterparts. As the department could not prove an association between diphtheria immunization and poliomyelitis, they advised medical officers to continue with the anti-diphtheria immunization campaign.[97]

By 1952, almost 60 per cent of pre-school children in the state presented to local health authority immunization schemes on an annual basis, although this figure fluctuated wildly from district to district. Following a similar pattern to that outlined in previous chapters, Cork city registered the highest coverage with 93 per cent of the pre-school population treated, followed by Louth at 90 per cent and Monaghan at 82 per cent. In Monaghan, county medical officer, Dr P. J. Deery, stated that anti-diphtheria immunization was so successful in his district that no case had occurred there for several years and that infectious disease in general had declined so much that the fever hospitals at Monaghan and Carrickmacross closed in 1954.[98] Dublin health authority returns showed 44 per cent coverage of the pre-school population, far lower than the national average. The meagre 19 per cent coverage in Limerick city demonstrated that immunization services available there had not kept pace with national developments. The ardent opposition to state medicine mounted by Limerick's municipal medical officer, Dr James McPolin, may explain this somewhat.[99] Of the 34 diphtheria cases reported nationally during 1954, 27 occurred in Dublin, and all five diphtheria fatalities that ensued also occurred in Dublin.[100] This trend continued in 1955 when 95 per cent of all diphtheria cases and 13 of 14 case fatalities occurred in Dublin city.[101] The *Irish Times* contextualized

---

96 W. J. McLeod, 'Poliomyelitis and diphtheria immunization in Belfast', *British Medical Journal* (7 April 1951), 736–38.

97 Department of Health, *Report 1950–51* (Dublin, 1952), 43. Notwithstanding the findings in Ireland, concerns relating to the association between immunization and poliomyelitis continued in England. For example, see, James Grant, 'Post-inoculation poliomyelitis', *British Medical Journal* (11 July 1953); Geffen and Tracy, 'Poliomyelitis in children under 6 months in England and Wales during 1950', *BMJ* (22 August 1953).

98 'County leads work in diphtheria immunization', *Irish Times*, 30 June 1956.

99 Department of Health, *Report 1952–53* (Dublin, 1954), Appendix 2, 60.

100 Department of Health, *Report 1953–54* (Dublin, 1955), 55.

101 'Diphtheria is still a child-killer', *Irish Times*, 26 November 1955.

these figures thus: 'Almost as many children have died from diphtheria in the city of Dublin as succumbed to the same cause last year in the whole of Britain, with its teeming population of fifty million people'.[102] Every diphtheria fatality in Dublin occurred in an unimmunized child: suggesting that Dublin's immunization services remained 'spasmodic and inconsistent'.[103]

In response, the Department of Health urged health authorities in general and those in Dublin in particular, to arrange for systematic follow up in homes where a written invitation to parents to have their children immunized failed to elicit a response. Furthermore, the department directed medical inspectors to ascertain if some features of immunization services organized by health authorities deterred parents from availing of it, and to remedy such shortcomings if revealed. Although a subsequent publicity drive in 1955 elicited a 'rush for immunization' late in the year,[104] incidence of the disease maintained an upward trend, driven almost exclusively by increased notifications in Dublin city. Of 229 cases notified for the year, Dublin provided 211, representing 92 per cent of diphtheria cases recorded in the state. Of the 16 case fatalities, 12 occurred in Dublin, representing 75 per cent of all diphtheria related fatalities.[105]

Addressing a gathering in County Dublin, in 1955, Minister for Health, T. F. O'Higgins, castigated parents who neglected to present their children for immunization treatment and asserted that they were not only 'failing in their duty as parents' but also 'failing in their duty as citizens'. Minister Higgins continued:

Ten years ago diphtheria was widespread. An intensive immunization campaign contributed largely to what seemed to be its virtual disappearance in a few years. Time and time again, however, the highest medical authorities told us that this happy state of affairs would continue only as long as the level of immunization in the community was kept up. Their warnings were unheeded by large numbers, and last year and again this year, we had unhappy evidence that the disease had not disappeared.[106]

Despite the existence of a regularized and systematic national anti-diphtheria programme, central health lamented that diphtheria continued to demand

102 'Diphtheria's mounting toll', *Irish Times*, 10 December 1955.
103 Department of Health, *Report 1955–56* (Dublin, 1957), 50.
104 'Immunization drive keeps clinics busy', *Irish Times*, 10 December 1955.
105 Department of Health, *Report 1956–57* (Dublin, 1958), 41.
106 'Parents could defeat dangerous diseases', *Irish Times*, 20 June 1956.

special attention from health authorities, particularly in Dublin.[107] By
the mid-1950s, more pressing public health issues in the shape of
tuberculosis, measles, whooping cough (pertussis), and poliomyelitis taxed
the resources of health authorities, particularly those resources relating to
disease prevention. While continued incidence or recrudescence of these
diseases urged increasing numbers of parents to submit their children for
immunization treatment, however, it was doctors in private practice, as
opposed to public health doctors, who noted the trend towards immunization.[108] In the latter half of the 1950s, general practitioners increasingly
reported that parents were contacting them to seek information not only
about diphtheria but also about the full scale of immunization services
available, including those services relating to the control of tuberculosis,
whooping cough, and smallpox.[109] One doctor observed: 'Previously it
was the kind of thing that you had to suggest [...] however, the need for
such suggestions seems to be disappearing. More and more parents are
looking for advice because of the publicity that this matter has received.
There is a great awareness of the need for having it done and it is having
a very good effect'.[110]

   The Department of Health bemoaned 'the inability or reluctance of
some [private] doctors' to furnish returns of immunization work done. This
made it impossible for local or central health authorities to make an accurate
assessment of the 'vaccinal or immunizational state of the population, or
particular groups thereof'.[111] Notwithstanding, by the beginning of the
1960s diphtheria rates in the Republic of Ireland fell to such negligible
numbers that the disease no longer featured as a standalone cause of death
in the annual statistical record.[112] Five diphtheria fatalities in non-immunized
children recorded during 1964 prompted then Minister for Health Donogh
O'Malley to issue a warning against complacency in regard to anti-diphtheria
immunization; cautioning that 'failure to have a child immunised may cost
its life and this is an onus that rests on parents and guardians'.[113] While the
majority of health districts were diphtheria free from the mid-1950s, the last
recorded case, which also proved to be the last recorded diphtheria fatality in

107 Department of Health, *Report 1957–58* (Dublin, 1959), 45. 'Apathy in diphtheria
     prevention', *Irish Times*, 16 January 1957. 'Slow response to diphtheria appeal', *Irish
     Times*, 4 April 1957.
108 'More seek protection against diphtheria', *Irish Times*, 29 May 1956.
109 *Irish Times*, 29 May 1956.
110 *Irish Times*, 29 May 1956.
111 Dáil Éireann, *Select committee on the health services* (1962), Chapter 1, Infectious disease
     service, 8.
112 Central Statistics Office, *Report on vital statistics 1964*, xx.
113 'A diphtheria warning to parents', *Irish Times*, 23 February 1966.

the state, occurred in 1967, 40 years after anti-diphtheria immunization had proven its efficacy in Dundalk.

By the mid-1960s, anti-diphtheria immunization was routinely carried out by means of a combined diphtheria/pertussis or diphtheria/tetanus/pertussis antigen, available free of charge at local dispensaries, public health clinics, and in schools. In addition, the Department of Health continued to supply diphtheria prophylactic free of charge to private practitioners on condition that they furnished returns of immunization work carried out with the material supplied.[114] The National BCG Committee expanded the national immunization programme to include anti-tuberculosis BCG vaccination, undertaken in the main by the health authority's medical staff, chiefly through the school medical service, and in a small number of areas on behalf of the health authority.[115] Vaccination against poliomyelitis was provided free of charge to persons aged between six months and 40 years, pregnant mothers, and 'certain classes at special risk', at centres supervised by a chief medical officer and his assistants, and a free vaccination service against smallpox continued at dispensaries and clinics.[116] The Irish Medical Association's submission to Dáil Éireann, requesting that family doctors, and not public health authorities, should oversee all immunization and vaccination procedures, was undermined somewhat by the question of remuneration. Central health determined that the discouraging effect of payment between patient and doctor would only serve to terminate the national immunization programme in its infancy, and rejected the proposal on that basis.

114 *Select committee on health services* (1962), 6–7.
115 See Margaret Ó hÓgartaigh, 'Dr Dorothy Price and the elimination of childhood tuberculosis', in Joost Augusteijn (ed.), *Ireland in the 1930s. New perspectives* (Dublin, 1999).
116 *Select committee on health services* (1962), 6–7.

Conclusion

This book is a significant addition to the history of medicine and health in twentieth-century Ireland. It charts the origins of childhood immunization in Ireland. It identifies the diverse factors which supported or obstructed the introduction of active immunization, and examines the rationale underpinning them. It highlights the centrality of municipal medical officers of health: their role in incepting and supervising local preventive public health initiatives in the face of popular resistance, and the uncooperative, and at times obstructionist stance adopted by the wider medical community.

In the 1920s, active immunization was a radical new public health intervention, widely considered to be in its experimental stage. It was rejected by government and by the medical community in Britain on that basis. The question then is why health authorities in the Irish Free State felt compelled to embark on such a largely untried intervention?

The study demonstrates that despite the distinct absence of diphtheria from the statistical record, the disease was rampant, and at times the most fatal of all childhood diseases in Ireland. Medical and popular ignorance as to the cause, nature, and treatment of diphtheria, combined with issues relating to nomenclature, and the reluctance of local authorities to have what was perceived as a new public health threat listed on their health reports, conspired to effectively obscure the true prevalence of diphtheria in Ireland. Such obfuscation simply allowed diphtheria to thrive and propagate, cloaked by doctors and local authorities unable or unwilling to intervene. Furthermore, diphtheria failed to feature prominently in the statistical record because there was no compulsion on local authorities to submit district reports of infectious diseases. Where national statistics are available, they are compiled from reports returned on a voluntary basis and at the discretion of local health authorities. This suggests that historians of health must approach the statistical data with some caution as the method of disease notification in nineteenth-century Ireland produced what can only be regarded as a partial and largely unreliable record.

Interpreting the statistical record is again confounded since the incidence of diphtheria in the Free State appears to increase substantially immediately following the introduction of anti-diphtheria immunization. A reliance on statistical data alone might lead an observer to suggest that active immunization failed to make any impact on the incidence of diphtheria in the state, or, taken a step further, the statistics may be appropriated to suggest that there was a link between the introduction of active immunization and an apparent rise in the numbers of diphtheria cases recorded. While the statistical record relating to the years immediately following the introduction of active immunization is a more accurate picture of the prevalence of diphtheria in the Free State, the significant increase can be explained by the rollout of full-time medical officers during the years 1928 to 1936 and a reflection of a more systematic method of notification employed by them.

The successful implementation of active immunization in New York and other North American cities was monitored with great interest by public health authorities worldwide. Graham Forbes's review of the New York intervention, and his comparison with preventive efforts to control diphtheria in Britain, aroused considerable interest in Ireland and Britain. Although active immunization was not readily accepted in Britain, the first independent Irish government was a strong advocate for the introduction of this new public health intervention. This initiative has previously been obscured by a historiography focused on civil war politics and issues of state building largely unconcerned with population health. Historical appraisals of the Cumann na nGaedheal administrations tend to lean towards a verdict suggesting a somewhat conservative tenure, and that government policy was dictated to a large extent by the British stance on any given issue. However, in the area of health reform, Cosgrave's governments were radical, progressive, and acted independently of decisions taken by their British counterparts. In this sense, and most possibly due to the influence of the American example, Ireland was ahead of Britain and much of Europe in adopting and implementing childhood immunization.

Engagement with local health records offers a new perspective on the history of medicine and health in Ireland. The records created by municipal medical officers of health have not featured prominently in Irish health histories to date. The reports compiled by Jack Saunders, Chief Superintendent Medical Officer to Cork City, 1929–57, place Cork city on the European frontline of the bacteriological revolution. Cork was the site of the first mass immunization scheme ever undertaken in Ireland and Britain and Saunders's intervention is a prime example of how a local initiative influenced national and international developments This programme was pursued with such zeal by the local medical officer that his efforts earned the city international recognition as 'the most immunized city in Europe'; it served as a model for public health doctors not only in Ireland, but in Britain also. Although Saunders's success in Cork exerted some pressure on Dublin's health authorities to tackle diphtheria, the records expose anti-diphtheria efforts in the capital as a miserly, haphazard, and ultimately unsuccessful intervention.

This study parallels work undertaken by Levene et al, Gorsky, and Welshman which independently confirm that municipal medicine in interwar Britain did not evolve in a uniform manner: findings which can also be readily identified in an Irish context. Comparative analysis of Cork and Dublin demonstrates that the public health response to diphtheria was not pursued with the same vigour in both localities. As has been confirmed in the British context, the success or otherwise of local initiatives in Ireland greatly relied on the personality of the supervising medical officer in each locality and was directly related to the level of enthusiasm which they brought to bear on any given public health intervention. The hands-on, and zealous, nature of the intervention supervised by Jack Saunders in Cork earned him international recognition as a leading field immunologist. Conversely, the supervising medical officer in Dublin, Matt Russell, was content to shirk his responsibility to address the presence of endemic diphtheria in Dublin by employing a part-time medical officer to oversee a very limited, and somewhat frugal, immunization scheme. Similarly, analysis of anti-diphtheria interventions, or the lack thereof, in Dundalk and Limerick serve to further highlight the disparity between levels of health service provision attendant on the attitudes of supervising medical officers in these localities.

Engagement with local health sources has also exposed an international controversy. The records reveal a somewhat dubious association between Irish medical officers of health and the British pharmaceutical company, Burroughs Wellcome Ltd, who supplied experimental anti-diphtheria prophylactics for testing on children in Irish residential institutions and among the general child population in Ireland. This association sits analogously within a historiography concerned with a prolonged separatist struggle against British imperialism, and a focus on the 'economic war' which strained Anglo-Irish relations in the post-independence period. Despite the protectionist economic policies adopted by the Fianna Fáil administration from 1932, Ireland remained heavily reliant on imported, and mainly British, anti-diphtheria prophylactics. There is some evidence to suggest that an Irish produced anti-diphtheria prophylactic developed by Ray O'Meara and Christopher McSweeney was due to come on the market in the late 1930s,[1]

---

1 Henry Moore, 'Dublin doctors triumph: New serum a great advance', *Irish Times*, 16 December 1940. See also, 'New diphtheria serum: Belfast committee and Dublin discovery', *Irish Times*, 18 December 1940.

in the wake of the Ring College controversy, however, there is little evidence to suggest that this ever came to fruition.[2]

The study addresses the perennial public health debate surrounding active immunization pertaining to the rights of the individual versus the pursuit of communal health. In relation to the Burroughs Wellcome-sponsored vaccine trials in Ireland, the rights of the most vulnerable section of Irish society, institutional children in state care, were clearly side-lined, not only in the pursuit of communal welfare, but also to satisfy the scientific curiosity and commercial interests of Burroughs Wellcome. This aspect of the study became the focus of national and international media attention in June 2014 and the controversial nature of the findings was instrumental in influencing Ireland's Department of Children and Youth Affairs to set up of a Commission of Investigation to examine historical issues relating to mother-and-baby homes, and vaccine trials conducted in Irish residential institutions.

Although the issue of Burroughs Wellcome-sponsored vaccine trials in Ireland has surfaced in the past, this study reveals that the practice was far more prevalent than previously known. The ill-fated Laffoy Commission,[3] set up to investigate claims that 245 children were subjected to vaccine trials in three children's institutions in 1962, 1971, and 1973 was abandoned after a successful Supreme Court challenge was taken by one of the doctors involved in the trials. A subsequent award-winning investigation undertaken by the Irish national broadcaster, RTÉ,[4] contained a statement from the successors of Burroughs Wellcome, GlaxoSmithKline, asserting that one further vaccine trial was undertaken, and had occurred during the 1970s. However, it is clear that Burroughs Wellcome-sponsored vaccine trials began at a much earlier period than was previously known and a focus on one single prophylactic has revealed that at least 2,051 children were subjected to vaccine trials in more than 22 institutions in the Free State and Wales between 1930 and 1935. In addition, the evidence suggests that up to 40,000 children among the general child population were unwittingly administered an experimental Burroughs Wellcome anti-diphtheria prophylactic before it was issued commercially in Britain.

2 Documentary sources relating to Christopher McSweeney and his work with Ray O'Meara to produce the 'Anti B' anti-diphtheria prophylactic at Cork Street Hospital, Dublin, have recently been acquired by the Royal College of Physicians Ireland. At the time of writing these documentary sources are being catalogued and have not been made available to researchers.

3 In June 2001, the Commission to Inquire into Child Abuse was given power to create a separate 'Vaccines Module' to investigate three known vaccine trials which came to light in 1997.

4 RTÉ, Primetime, 'Anatomy of a scandal': Produced by Tanya Sillem and Katie Hannon. (First screened on 6 October 2011) was awarded 'Story of the Year' at the GSK sponsored Irish Medical Media Awards 2012.

Burroughs Wellcome-sponsored vaccine trials were undertaken on a systematic basis in Ireland in the mid-twentieth century. The administrators of the institutions involved gave their full consent to the trials which include state-run orphanages, mother-and-baby homes, an institute for the deaf and dumb, and children's hospitals. Although some commentators assert that religious congregations who ran the residential institutions involved received remuneration for their consent, there is no evidence to substantiate such claims.

It is more likely that resident medical officers informed religious orders in charge of such institutions that children under their care were being treated under a general immunization scheme. In fact, evidence suggests parents and guardians of children in public, private, and institutional spheres involved in Burroughs Wellcome-sponsored trials were kept in the dark with regard to the highly experimental and potentially lethal nature of the vaccines administered to children in their care. While commentators are quick to judge religious congregations, there has been little or no attention given to the medical and scientific communities who facilitated trials. These include state-paid institutional medical officers, state-paid municipal and county medical officers, and state-paid academics. In short, any future investigation should not focus solely on religious congregations, but must consider the role of the medical and scientific community also, and the salaried medical personnel who bore ultimate responsibility for the health and wellbeing of children in state care.

Vaccine trials now in the public domain were conducted before the introduction of the Control of Clinical Trials Act 1987, and in this sense, they were not illegal or unlawful. They were governed by what amounted to little more than a 'utilitarian ethic', where the benefits to the many from human experimentation was considered as justification for the lack of a full appreciation of the rights of trial subjects, particularly in regard to obtaining their consent for participation in research. However, there are further ethical issues to be explored. British pharmaceutical companies conducted vaccine trials on children in Ireland because they were debarred from doing so under legislation in Britain. Who decided that Irish children were creatures of lesser standing, bereft of the rights and special protection afforded their British counterparts? Who decided that vulnerable Irish children in state care should be exposed to the unnecessary risks associated with experimental vaccines? Were institutional 'guardians' properly placed to allow children to be used as 'experimental material' in vaccine trials? If so, was their decision made in the best interest of the children or was it to satisfy scientific and commercial concerns?[5]

5 Michael Dwyer, 'Vaccine Trials: Dark chapter that needs answers', *Irish Examiner*, 1 December 2014.

Issues of professionalization and medical ethics are further explored by revisiting the Ring College immunization disaster. Although the existing historiography relating to the incident is brief and generally ill-informed, there is consensus among existing studies that a phial of live tuberculosis was accidentally issued by Burroughs Wellcome for use in an anti-diphtheria scheme in County Waterford. Although a High Court ruling failed to apportion blame to Burroughs Wellcome, historians have insisted on implicating the company in the tragedy. This study produces new evidence contradicting this tradition and suggests that the local doctor was culpable, aided and abetted by prominent physicians who mounted a conspiracy of criminal proportions to protect their beleaguered colleague.

This suggestion is underpinned by the introduction and exploration of new and previously unexplored sources unearthed at the Wellcome Archives and Manuscripts Collection, London, which bring a new interpretation to bear on events surrounding the Ring College affair. While the cause of the immunization accident at Ring may never be known, this new evidence suggests that the local attending physician Daniel McCarthy and the college principal Séamus Ó hEocha went to great lengths to conceal the severity of the infections experienced by children in their care from their parents and although tubercular infections were confirmed in every case this information was not made public. It is clear from a letter sent by the university bacteriologist William O'Donovan to McCarthy that the prominent surgeon Patrick Kiely had suggested that the Ring incident should be presented in terms which closely echoed events surrounding an immunization disaster in Lübeck, Germany, where a laboratory-based mishap and its consequences were still fresh in the public memory. The result: that the actions of one doctor could undermine an international public health intervention. This study presents the Ring incident as a historical precedent which closely mirrors events surrounding the more recent Andrew Wakefield MMR controversy. In this sense, this aspect of the study demonstrates the importance of examining historical vaccine controversies, and a community's past experiences with vaccines in general, so that vaccine hesitancy may be better understood today.

A re-consideration of the historical significance of the Ring College immunization disaster combined with revelations surrounding Burroughs Wellcome-sponsored trials in Ireland challenges Jane Lewis's findings in her study relating to the rollout of anti-diphtheria immunization in Britain. Lewis's study determined that the delayed introduction of active immunization in Britain was, in the main, due to economic considerations; however, her study fails to take cognizance of the implications attendant on the significant transnational interests at play in the interwar period. The Ring incident received global media attention and was watched closely by medical and political commentators in Britain. It is highly unlikely that the negative repercussions attendant on the Ring affair were limited to Ireland and it is my contention that this immunization disaster was a major influence on the decision to delay the rollout of active immunization in Britain.

Thomas McKeown argues that the growth of populations since the eighteenth-century has little to do with targeted public health interventions and more to do with broad-based efforts to distribute social, political, and economic resources particularly in relation to improved standards of living, better housing, better nutrition, and increased natural immunity. The 'McKeown thesis' has generated much scholarship which variously support and criticize his conclusions, and the associated themes have been vigorously argued particularly in relation to the demise of tuberculosis.[6] In relation to diphtheria, and I contend that the same holds true for many other infectious diseases, environmental and socioeconomic factors had little bearing on the incidence of diphtheria in the pre-vaccine age. It struck down poverty-stricken tenement bound children in New York, London, and Dublin as well as the august children of the European monarchs housed in palatial grandeur. This is because the specific diphtheria germ does not exist in the environment but in the individual. If we consider that the campaign to control diphtheria in Ireland succeeded in achieving its goal during the 1950s – a period regarded as being 'a miserable decade [...] marked by a series of panic fiscal measures'[7] – then it must be reasonable to suggest that the control of diphtheria in Ireland was achieved solely through a medical intervention in the shape of active immunization.

It is virtually impossible to discuss the broader determinants of health without some historical perspective. Current public health policies are not created, nor do they operate in a vacuum; however, public health students are often taken aback at the scale of improvements in the health of populations over relatively short time scales and this is relevant to reflections on underlying driving forces. Students are regularly surprised at how historical perspective highlights the extent to which the same debates and issues recur, albeit in modified form, in virtually every generation: issues such as the state versus the individual, the health of the community versus the rights of the individual, and issues relating to the safety of new drugs and vaccines.

The success or otherwise of immunization campaigns is determined by levels of public confidence; however, safety concerns propagated through

6 See Thomas McKeown, *The modern rise of populations* (London, 1976), Bryder, Condrau, Worboys, 'Tuberculosis and its histories: Then and now', in *Tuberculosis then and now: Perspectives on the history of an infectious disease* (London, 2010).

7 Cormac O'Grada, *A rocky road: The Irish economy since the 1920s* (Manchester, 1997), 25. See also; Tom Garvin, *Preventing the future: Why was Ireland so poor for so long?* (Dublin, 2004).

social, and news media, continually serve to reinforce common misconceptions about vaccines, and repeatedly undermine confidence in active immunization. Debate surrounding the safety and role of childhood immunization is of course necessary, but much of this discussion has taken place in the absence of a full understanding of historical factors which have determined current polarized views. In the West, active immunization is becoming a victim of its own success: its enduring achievement has relegated the status of childhood disease to a level of relative obscurity. Many diseases have been consigned to history, but so too have the horrors and mass fatalities once associated with them. The success of childhood immunization has meant that entire populations have never encountered diseases which vaccines actively prevent and there has been a societal shift to focusing more on the dangers associated with the needle and the vaccine, rather than the risk posed by the disease itself.

The rollout of immunization schemes in the early twentieth century presented parents and public health authorities with difficult decisions, which in many respects mirror difficult decisions faced by parents, doctors, and public health workers today. The success of the anti-diphtheria program in Ireland has meant that no child has endured the adverse and frequently fatal consequences of contracting this once 'most deadly disease of childhood' and no Irish parent has suffered the loss of a child to diphtheria in the last fifty years. However, after such a prolonged absence, a case of diphtheria was notified in Ireland during 2015 and the National Health Protection Surveillance Centre confirmed that another case notified in 2016. Both cases occurred in adults and were non-fatal; however, this is a stark reminder that diphtheria has not been eradicated. It is controlled by vaccines, but is waiting to re-emerge. Science has not conquered diphtheria, it has merely contained it, and the duration of this containment relies on the veracity of our vaccines and the continued willingness of parents to submit children to the national immunization program.

Bibliography

Archives

Key to archive material:
CC&CA Cork City and County Archives
CCCLS Cork City Library Local Studies Department
CSFH Royal College of Physicians Ireland
NAI National Archives of Ireland, Dublin
WA Wellcome Archives and Manuscript Collection, London

CC&CA, CP/C/CM/PH/A/30. Letter from Dr. D. J. Carroll, Medical Officer of Health for Cork County Borough to the Hon. Secretary and chairman, Cork Fever Hospital, July 1927.
CC&CA, CP/C/CM/PH/A/30. Letter from Minister of Local Government and Public Health: No. M.53621/1926.
CC&CA, CP/C/CM/PH/A/30. Letter from Sir John Scott to Donal Carroll, Chief Superintendent Medical Officer of Health for Cork County Borough, dated 6 July 1927.
CC&CA, CP/C/CM/PH/A/30. This file contains the weekly records of the incidence of infectious disease in Cork city, compiled by the municipal public health department since 1878.
CCCLS/352.4. J. C. Saunders, *Report of the Medical Officer of Health for the years 1930–47, and 1951–54.*
CSFH RCPI. Cork Street Fever Hospital and Cherry Orchard Hospital Papers.
CSFH/3. Medical Superintendents Papers.
CSFH/3/1/2/7. Development of diphtheria and scarlet fever vaccines.
CSFH/3/1/2/7. Letter from Richard O'Brien to Christopher McSweeney, 22 December 1933.
CSFH/3/1/2/7. Letter from Richard O'Brien to Christopher McSweeney, 19 February 1934.
CSFH/3/1/2/7. Letter from Richard O'Brien to Christopher McSweeney, 4 February 1935.
NAI HLTH Bl 32/14. Diphtheria Vaccination Statistics 1948–68.
NAI HLTH Bl 32/26. Public Health Circular 10/40 1948.
NAI HLTH Bl 32/37. Improved Prophylactics.
NAI HLTH Bl 32/43. General Immunization Schemes.

NAI HLTH B1 36/10. Burroughs Wellcome Licences, Vol. i 1939–50; Vol. ii 1950–56; Vol. iii 1951–53.

NAI HLTH B1 36/40. C. J. McSweeney Licence No. 40, 1936–38.

NAI HLTH B1/32/16. Diphtheria Prophylactics, Vol. i 1943–44; Vol. ii 1945–52.

NAI HLTH B23/22. Immunization against Diphtheria Vol. i.

NAI HLTH B29/24. Ring College 1935–48.

NAI HLTH B33/20. Cork County Borough 1943–44.

NAI HLTH B34/63. Dublin County Borough, Vol. i 1930–43; Vol. ii 1939–50; Vol. iii 1949–53.

WA/B/13556083. James A. Harbison, *Report of the Medical Officer of Health, City of Dublin, for the years 1948, 1951, 1953–54.*

WA/B/13556083. John B. O'Regan, *Report of the City Medical Officer, City of Dublin, for the year 1955.*

WA/B/13556083. Matthew J. Russell, *Report on the state of public health in the City of Dublin for the years 1929, 1931,1933–38, 1940, 1944.*

WA/B/13556083. Morgan P. Crowe (Acting MOH), *Report on the state of public health in the City of Dublin for the year 1947.*

WA/B/13556794. J. C. Saunders, *Report of the Medical Officer of Health for the years 1948–50.*

WA/PP/JRH/A/75. Box 8, Robert Percy McDonnell, Notes on Dungarvan outbreak.

WA/PRL/HP/Sub/29/10. William O'Donovan, Private Preliminary Report No. 4243.

WA/PRL/HP/Sub/33/5. Daniel McCarthy, Report on diphtheria immunization in Ring College, 23 February 1937.

WA/PRL/HP/Sub/33/5. J. C. Saunders, Letter to Henry Parish, 27 February 1937.

WA/PRL/HP/Sub/33/5. J. C. Saunders, Letter to John Trevan, 1 March 1937.

WA/PRL/HP/Sub/33/5. J. C. Saunders, Letter to R. A. O'Brien, 23 February 1937.

WA/PRL/HP/Sub/33/5. John Trevan, Letter to J. C. Saunders, 25 February 1937.

WA/WF/L/02/27. Henry Parish, Accident at Ring, near Dungarvan, Co. Waterford.

WA/WF/L/02/27. Richard O'Brien, General Notes.

WA/WF/L/02/27. Richard O'Brien, I. F. S. Professor Bigger, 17 May 1937.

WA/WF/L/02/27. Richard O'Brien, I. F. S.-Ring, Confidential Report.

WA/WF/L/02/27. Richard O'Brien, Memorandum-I. F. S. Ring, 29 May 1937.

WF/L/02/09, J. J. Horgan, Letter to Markby, Stewart and Wadesons, 1 November 1937.

WF/L/02/09, J. J. Horgan, Letter to Markby, Stewart, and Wadesons, Solicitors, 1 July 1937.

WF/L/02/09. Henry Parish, Letter to J. J. Horgan, 28 June 1937.

WF/L/02/09. J. C. Saunders, Letter to Henry Parish, 24 September 1937.

WF/L/02/09. J. J. Horgan to Henry Parish, 9 August 1937.

WF/L/02/09. J. J. Horgan, Letter to Henry Parish, 14 June 1937.

WF/L/02/09. J. J. Horgan, Letter to Henry Parish, 26 June 1937.

WF/L/02/09. J. J. Horgan, Letter to Henry Parish, 9 July 1937.

WF/L/02/09. J. J. Horgan, Letter to Markby, Stewart and Wadesons, 13 November 1937.

WF/L/02/09. J. J. Horgan, Letter to Markby, Stewart, and Wadesons, Solicitors, 14 June 1937.

WF/L/02/09. Letter from J. J. Horgan to Parish, 18 June 1937, letter from J. C. Saunders to Parish, 24 September 1937, and letter from J. J. Horgan to Markby, Stewart and Wadesons, 1 November 1937.

WF/L/02/14, R. P. McDonnell, Department of Local Government and Public Health, Letter to J. J. Horgan, 17 December 1938.

WF/L/02/14. J. J. Horgan, Letter to R. P. McDonnell, Department of Local Government and Public Health, 2 December 1938.

WF/L/02/14. List of children immunised against diphtheria in November 1936.

WF/L/02/14. Michael O'Donnell, Letter to J. J. Horgan, 19 January 1939.

WF/L/02/14. Michael O'Donnell, Letter to J. J. Horgan, 21 January 1939.

WF/L/02/14. Michael O'Donnell, Letter to J. J. Horgan, 28 January 1939.

WF/L/02/14. R. P. McDonnell, Department of Local Government and Public Health, Letter to J. J. Horgan, 9 December 1938.

WF/M/GB/01/37/01. Daniel McCarthy, Private and Confidential Report from Dr McCarthy to Department of Local Government and Public Health.

WF/M/GB/01/37/01. Henry Parish, Confidential Notes on visit to Cork.

WF/M/GB/01/37/01. J. J. Horgan, Interview with Nurse Elizabeth Denn, 8 October 1938.

WF/M/GB/01/37/1. Richard O'Brien, Notes on accident at Ring, 4 May 1937.

WF/M/H/08/10. Henry Parish, *The Wellcome Research Laboratories and immunization: A historical survey and personal memoir*, Chapters 7 to 9, c. 1970.

Official Publications

Dáil Éireann, *Select committee on the health services* (1962).

Department of Health, *Health Act, 1947* (Stationery Office, Dublin, 1947).

Department of Health, *Health progress 1947–1953* (Stationery Office, Dublin, 1953).

Department of Health, *Report on 3 Clinical Trials involving babies and children in institutional settings 1960/61, 1970 and 1973.*

Department of Health, *Reports 1945–58* (Stationery Office, Dublin).

Department of Local Government and Public Health, *Local Government Act 1925.*

Department of Local Government and Public Health, *Ministers and Secretaries (Amendment) Act, 1946.*

Department of Local Government and Public Health, *Reports, 1925–44,* (Stationery Office, Dublin).

Department of Local Government and Public Health, *The Public Health (Infectious Disease) Regulations, 1929, Amendment No. 4.*

Department of Local Government and Public Health, *The Therapeutic Substance Regulations*, dated July 25, 1931, made by the Joint Committee constituted by sec. 4 (1) of the Acts, S.R. and O. 1931, No. 633.

'Diphtheria immunization', *Great Britain, Parliament, House of Commons*, Vol. 343, 46, cc. 1937–8W, 16 February 1939.

Contemporary Newspapers and Periodicals

American Journal of Public Health
Anglo Celt
British Medical Journal
Connaught Telegraph
Cork Examiner
Dublin Journal of Medical Science
Dungarvan Observer
Irish Independent
Irish Journal of Medical Science
Irish Press
Irish Times
The Lancet
Medical History
Munster Express
Nenagh News
The Times
Tuam Herald

Contemporary Publications

'A fatality after diphtheria immunization', *British Medical Journal*, 5 June 1937, 1182–83.

Anderson, McLeod, et al, 'Starch fermentation by the "gravis" type of diphtheria', *The Lancet*, Vol. 221, No. 571 (11 February 1933), 293–95.

'An epidemic in New Ross', *British Medical Journal* (4 November 1911), 1226.

Armstrong, Charles, 'Post-vaccination encephalitis', *Annals of Internal Medicine*, Vol. 5. No. 3, (1 September 1931), 333–37.

Bailey, Ridley, 'Public health progress in the Queen's reign, 1837–1897: being the presidential address of the Midland Branch of the incorporated Society of Medical Officers of Health 1897', *LSE Selected Pamphlets* (1897), 24.

Banks H. Stanley, and A. J. Beale, 'Poliomyelitis and immunization against whooping cough and diphtheria', *British Medical Journal* (29 July 1950), 251–52.

Bernard, Walter, 'Diphtheria in Londonderry', *Dublin Journal of Medical Science*, Vol. 71, No. 5 (2 May 1881), 402–04.

Black, J. B., 'The accidental transmission of malaria through intravenous injections of op neoarsphenamine', *American Journal of Epidemiology*, 31, Section (2), (1940), 37–42.

Bosanquet, William C. and John Eyre, *Serums, vaccines and toxins in treatment and diagnosis* (London, Cassell & Co, 1909).

Bousfield, Guy, 'Diphtheria immunization', *British Medical Journal* (26 January 1935), 181.

Bradford Hill, A. and J. Knowelden, 'Inoculation and poliomyelitis: A statistical investigation in England and Wales in 1949', *British Medical Journal* (1 July 1950), 1–6.

Buchan, G. F., 'Society of Medical Officers of Health', *British Medical Journal* (24 October 1925), 751.

Budding, Mary E., 'Immunization and poliomyelitis', *British Medical Journal* (27 May 1950), 1273.

Butler, Stuyvesant and Samuel A. Levine, 'Diphtheria as a cause of late heart-block', *American Heart Journal*, Vol. 5, No. 5 (June 1930), 592–98.

Chesney, George, 'Alum-precipitated Toxoid in diphtheria immunization', *British Medical Journal* (1 February 1936), 208–09.

Collins, Selwyn, D., 'History and frequency of diphtheria immunizations and cases in 9,000 families', *Public Health Reports* (1896–1970), Vol. 51, No. 51 (18 December 1936), 1736–73.

Collis, W. R. F., 'Some facts and figures in relation to health in Dublin', *Irish Journal of Medical Science*, No. 173 (May 1940), 193–200.

Copeman, Sydney Monkton, 'A British Medical Association lecture on immunization against diphtheria, scarlet fever, and measles', *British Medical Journal*, Vol. 1, No. 3515 (19 May 1928), 833–35.

Creighton, Charles, *A history of epidemics in Britain, volume II, from the extinction of plague to the present time* (London, C. J. Lane & Sons, 1894).

Cruickshank, Robert, 'Poliomyelitis after immunization', *British Medical Journal* (13 May 1950), 1139.

Crum, Frederick S., 'A statistical study of diphtheria', *American Journal of Public Health*, Vol. VII, No. 5 (May 1917), 445.

Darnton, Marguerite, 'Immunization and poliomyelitis', *British Medical Journal* (24 June 1950), 1489.

Dickens, Charles (ed.), 'A grumble', *All the year round* (19 March 1864), 136–38.

Douglas, S. R. and Percival Hartley, 'The preparation of old tuberculin by the use of synthetic media with observations on its properties and stability'. *Tubercle*, 16 (1935), 105–13.

'Epidemic disease in Dublin', *British Medical Journal* (25 February 1911), 463.

Fitzgerald, J. G., 'Diphtheria toxoid as an immunizing agent', *Journal of the Canadian Medical Association*, Vol. 17, No. 5 (May 1927), 524–29.

Flaubert, Gustave, *L'éducation sentimentale* (Paris, Bréal, 2000).

Forbes, J. Graham, 'Diphtheria in London', *The Lancet*, Vol. 210, No. 5421 (9 July 1927), 203.

Forbes, J. Graham, 'Progress of diphtheria prevention; a survey and some results', *British Medical Journal* (18 December 1937), 1209.

Forbes, J. Graham, 'The problem of the diphtheria carrier in London children of school age', *Public Health*, XXXVI (1923), 323.

Forbes, J. Graham, *The prevention of diphtheria* (London, Medical Research Council, 1927).

Fothergill, John, *An account of the sore throat attended with ulcers* (London, C. Davis, 1754).

Gaffney, James C., 'A statistical study of the epidemiology and prevention of diphtheria in Dublin; Part I', *Irish Journal of Medical Science*, No. 208 (April 1943), 97–115.

Geffen, D. H., 'The incidence of paralysis occurring in London children within four weeks after immunization', *Medical Officer*, Vol. 83 (8 April 1950), 137–40.

Geffen, D. H., P. J. Hamilton, and S. M. Tracy, 'Poliomyelitis in children under 6 months in England and Wales during 1950', *British Medical Journal*, Vol. 2, No. 4833 (22 August 1953), 427–29.

Glenny, A. T., 'Insoluble precipitates in diphtheria and tetanus immunization', *British Medical Journal*, Vol. 2, No. 244 (16 August 1930), 244.

Godfrey, Edward, S., 'Study in the epidemiology of diphtheria in relation to active immunization of certain age groups', *American Journal of Public Health*, Vol. 22, No. 3 (March 1932), 237.

Grant, James, 'Post-inoculation poliomyelitis', *British Medical Journal*, Vol. 2, No. 4827 (11 July 1953), 66–70.

Greenhow, E. H., *On diphtheria* (New York, Bailliére Brothers, 1861).

Guthrie, C., J. Gilien, W. L. Moss, 'Diphtheria Bacillus Carriers', 2nd Communication, *Bulletin; John Hopkins Hospital*, No. 31 (1920), 388.

Hanley, Denis, 'Anti-diphtheria immunization', *Irish Journal of Medical Science*, Vol. 12, Issue 9 (September 1937), 578–85.

Hecker, J. F. C., *The epidemics of the Middle Ages* (London, G. Woodfall, 1844).

'Immunization against diphtheria', *British Medical Journal* (9 November 1935), 420, 908–09.

'International congress of microbiology', *British Medical Journal* (1 August 1936), 253–54.

'Ireland', *British Medical Journal* (16 January 1904), 158.

'Ireland', *British Medical Journal* (7 January 1911), 41.

'Ireland', *British Medical Journal* (1 July 1911), 47.

Leete, McLeod, Morrison, 'Diphtheria in Hull and its relation to bacteriological type', *The Lancet*, Vol. 22, No. 5751 (18 November1933), 1141–44.

'Lessons from the outbreak of diphtheria in the Grand Ducal family of Hesse-Darmstadt', *British Medical Journal* (4 January 1879), 15.

Letters, Patrick, 'Public Health and preventable disease in the counties of Cork, Kerry, and Waterford', *The Dublin Journal of Medical Science*, Vol. 107, No. 3 (1 March 1899), 181–89.

Loeffler, Frederick, 'The history of diphtheria', in G. H. F. Nuttall (ed.), *The bacteriology of diphtheria* (Cambridge, Cambridge University Press, 1908).

McCloskey, Bertram P., 'The relation of prophylactic inoculations to the onset of poliomyelitis', *The Lancet*, Vol. 255, No. 6606 (8 April 1950), 659–63.

McLeod, John, *Proceedings of the Royal Society of Medicine*, Vol. XXIX, July 1936, Section on Pathology.

McLeod, W. J., 'Poliomyelitis and diphtheria immunization in Belfast', *British Medical Journal* (7 April 1951), 736–38.

Macrobius, *Saturnalia*, 1, 10.

McSweeney, C. J., 'An evaluation of modern diphtheria prophylactics', *British Medical Journal* (19 January 1935), 103–05.

McSweeney, C. J., 'The prevention of diphtheria', Paper read before the Medical Society, University College Dublin, 3 December 1934.

McSweeney, C. J., 'The prevention of diphtheria', *Irish Journal of Medical Science'*, Vol. 10, No. 2 (February 1935), 76–81.

Martin, J. K., 'Local paralysis in children after injections', *Archives of Disease in Childhood*, Vol. 25, No. 121 (1950), 1–14.

Memoirs of the Medical Society of London, Volume I (London, Fry & Couchman, 1787).

'Mortality from diphtheria decreasing', *American Journal of Public Health*, Vol. 16, No. 6 (June 1926), 621.

Mouillot, Albert, 'On an outbreak of diphtheria', *Dublin Journal of Medical Science* (1 April 1887), 352–55.

Naughten, White, Foley, 'Prevention of diphtheria by the "one-shot" method using alum-precipitated toxoid', *British Medical Journal* (9 November 1935), 893.

Newsholme, Arthur, *Epidemic diphtheria: A research on the origin and spread of the disease from an international standpoint* (London, Sonnenschein, 1898).

O'Brien, Catherine, 'In Memoriam, Matthew John Russell', *Irish Journal of Medical Science* (April 1956), 190.

O'Brien, Catherine, *Annual report of the school medical service for the year ended 31st December 1944* (County Borough of Dublin, 1945).

O'Brien, R. A., 'Immunization in the prevention of specific fevers', *British Medical Journal* (20 October 1934), 712–14.

O'Brien, R. A., 'Schick test and subsequent active immunization', *Proceedings of the Royal Society of Medicine*, No. 15 (1922), 45–48.

O'Brien, R. A., 'The control of diphtheria and scarlet fever', *British Medical Journal* (8 September 1928), 712.

Oertel, J., 'The outbreak of diphtheria in the Grand Ducal family of Hesse-Darmstadt', *British Medical Journal* (11 January 1879), 36–39.

O'Leary, Mary M., 'A survey of the health of the Dublin school child', *Irish Journal of Medical Science* (April 1931), 155–61.

O'Meara, R. A. Q., 'The prevalence of diphtheria carriers among Dublin school children', *Irish Journal of Medical Science*, Vol. 6, No. 3 (March 1931), 125–33.

Parish, H. J., 'Immunization against diphtheria with Alum-Precipitated Toxoid (APT)', *British Medical Journal* (1 February 1936), 209–10.

Park, William and Abraham Zingher, 'Diphtheria immunity-natural, active and passive. Its determination by the Schick Test', *American Journal of Public Health*, Vol. 6, No. 5 (May 1916), 431.

Park, William and Abraham Zingher, 'The control of diphtheria', *American Journal of Public Health*, Vol. 13, No. 1 (January 1923), 26.

Park, William, 'Some important facts concerning active immunization against diphtheria', *American Journal of Diseases of Children*, Vol. 32, No. 5 (1926), 709–17.

Park, William, and Abraham Zingher, 'Diphtheria toxin-antitoxin and toxoid; a comparison', *American Journal of Public Health and the Nation's Health*, Vol. 22, No. 1 (January 1932), 7–16.

'Poliomyelitis after immunization', *British Medical Journal* (15 April 1950), 890–91.

Price, Dorothy, 'Tuberculosis in adolescents', *Irish Journal of Medical Science*, Vol. 14, No. 3 (1939), 124–29.

Railton, Thomas Carleton, 'The early symptoms of some of the infectious diseases (1890)', *LSE Selected Pamphlets*, 11–14.

'Report of the medical history of the attack of diphtheria in the Grand Ducal family at Hesse-Darmstadt', *British Medical Journal* (4 January 1879), 6.

Rutty, John, *Chronological history of the weather and seasons, and prevailing diseases in Dublin, during forty years* (London, Robertson & Roberts, 1770).

Saunders, J. C., 'Alum-Precipitated Toxoid in diphtheria prevention', *The Lancet*, Vol. 229, No. 5931 (1 May 1937), 1064–68.

Saunders, J. C., 'Alum-Toxoid as an immunising agent against diphtheria', *The Lancet*, Vol. 220, No. 5698 (12 November 1932), 1047–50.

Saunders, J. C., 'The occurrence of diphtheria in "immunised" persons', *Irish Journal of Medical Science*, Vol. 8, No. 11 (November 1933), 611–19.

Saunders, J. C., 'The reactions with alum-toxoid in diphtheria prophylaxes', *The Lancet*, Vol. 221, No. 5720 (15 April 1933), 791–96.

Saunders, J. C., 'The trend of diphtheria mortality in the Irish Free State', *Irish Journal of Medical Science* (September 1934), 520–26.

Saunders, J. C., *'Trends in diphtheria prophylaxis'*, Paper read before the Cork Clinical Society, 2 February 1935.

Sawyer, Robert, 'Diphtheria formol toxoid and the Moloney test', *The Lancet*, Vol. 226, No. 5836 (6 July 1935), 22.

Semple, Robert Hunter (trans), *Memoirs on diphtheria, from the writings of Bretonneau, Guersant, Trousseau, Bouchut, Empis, and Daviot* (London, James William Roche, 1859).

Short, Thomas, *A general chronological history of the air, weather, seasons, meteors, etc. In sundry places and different times more particularly for the space of 250 years*, Volume II (London, Longman & Millar, 1749).

Slade, Daniel, D., *Diphtheria: its nature and treatment, an account of the history of its prevalence in various countries* (Philadelphia, Collins, 1864).

Sorsby, Max, 'A note on diphtheria immunization in London', *British Medical Journal* (1 October 1938), 701–03.

St John Gogarty, Oliver, 'The need of medical inspection of school children in Ireland', *The Irish Review*, Vol. 2, No. 13 (March 1912), 14.

Symes, William Langford, 'On the mortality of children in Ireland (1886–1896)', *Transactions of the Royal Academy of Medicine in Ireland*, Vol. 16, No. 1 (December 1898), 381–94.

Symes, William Langford, 'On the symptoms or phenomena formerly known as Croup; the diseases which produce them; and the clinical significance of the varied allied affections embraced by the term', *Transactions of the Royal Academy of Medicine in Ireland*, Vol. 18, No. 1 (December 1900), 68–69.

'The Lübeck disaster', *American Journal of Public Health*, Vol. 21, No. 3 (March 1931), 282.

'Toxoid and toxin-antitoxin in diphtheria immunization', *British Medical Journal*, Vol. 2, No. 3574 (6 July 1929), 22–23.

Trall, R. T., *Diphtheria: its nature, history, causes, prevention, and treatment on hygienic principles with a resúme of the various practices of the medical profession* (New York, R. T. Trall & Co, 1862).

Tzen, Dzen, and Chang, 'Report on accident following the use of diphtheria toxin-antitoxin mixture', *China Medical Journal*, No. 41 (1927), 412–23.

Underwood, E. Ashford, '"One-shot" Immunization against diphtheria', *British Medical Journal* (23 June 1934), 1140.

Underwood, E. Ashworth, 'The diphtheria toxoid-reaction (Moloney) test: its applications and significance', *Journal of Hygiene*, Vol. 35, No. 4 (December 1935), 449–75.

Von Sholly, Anna and Harriet Wilcox, 'A contribution to the statistics of the presence of diphtheria bacilli in apparently normal throats', *Journal of Infectious Diseases*, Vol. 4 (1907), 337–46.

Walpole, Horace, *Letters of Horace Walpole, Earl of Oxford, to Sir Horace Mann*, Volume I (London, Richard Bentley, 1843).

Wells, D. M., Graham, H. and Havens, L. C., 'Diphtheria toxoid precipitated with alum: its preparation and advantages', *American Journal of Public Health*, Nations Health, Vol. 22, No. 6 (June 1932), 648–50.

Secondary Sources

Adams, Francis (trans), *The extant works of Aretaeus, The Cappadocian* (Boston, Millford House, 1972).

Adler, N. R, Mahony, A. and Friedman, N. D. 'Diphtheria: forgotten, but not gone', *Internal Medicine Journal*, Vol. 43, No. 2 (February 2013), 206–10.

Barrington, Ruth, *Health, medicine, and politics in Ireland 1900–1970* (Dublin, Institute of Public Administration, 1987).

Berridge, Virginia, 'History in public health: who needs it?', *The Lancet*, Vol. 356, No. 9245, (2 December 2000), 1923–25.

Berridge, Virginia, 'History in the public health tool kit', *Journal of Epidemiology and Community Health*, Vol. 55 (2001), 611–12.

Berridge, Virginia, 'History matters? History's role in health policy making', *Medical History*, Vol. 52, No. 3 (May 2008), 311–26.

Berridge, Virginia, Martin Gorsky and Alex Mold, *Public health in history* (Maidenhead, Open University Press, 2011).

Beyazova, Sahin, and Ben S. Yucel, 'Age specific diphtheria immunity', in Ben S. Wheeler (ed.), *Trends in diphtheria research* (New York, Nova Science, 2006).

Bonah, Christian and Phillippe Menut, 'BCG vaccination, the Lübeck scandal, and the Reichsrichtlinien', in V. Roelcke and G. Maoi (eds), *Twentieth century ethics in human subjects research; historical perspectives on values, practices, and regulations* (München, Franz Steiner Verlag, 2004).

Brandt, Allan M., 'Emerging themes in the history of medicine', *The Millbank Quarterly*, Vol. 69, No. 2 (1991): 199–214.

Brieger, G. H., 'The historiography of medicine', in Bynam, W. F. and Porter, R. (eds), *Companion encyclopaedia of the history of medicine* (Routledge, London, 1993), Vol. 1, 24.

Bristow, Adrian F. et al, 'Standardization of biological medicines: the first hundred years, 1900–2000', *Notes and Records of The Royal Society*, Vol. 60. No. 3 (22 September 2006), 271–89.

Browne, Noel, *Against the tide* (Dublin, Gill & Macmillan, 1986).

Brunton, Deborah, 'The problems of implementation: the failure and success of public vaccination against smallpox in Ireland, 1840–1873' in *Medicine, disease and the state in Ireland, 1650–1940* (Cork, Cork University Press, 1999).

Bryder, Linda, Flurin Condrau and Michael Worboys, 'Tuberculosis and its histories: Then and now', in *Tuberculosis then and now: Perspectives on the history of an infectious disease* (London, Montreal & Kingston, 2010).

Carroll, Lydia, *In the fever king's preserve; Sir Charles Cameron and the Dublin slums* (Dublin, A & A Farmar, 2011).

Cartwright, Anthony, 'Medicines regulation', in O'Grady, J., Dobbs-Smith, I., Walsh, N. and Spencer, M. (eds), *Medicines, medical devices and the law* (Cambridge, Cambridge University Press, 1999).

Castellani, C., 'La "Lettera medica" di Martino Ghisi relative alla 'Istoria delle angine epidemiche', *Rivista di storia della medicina*, No. 2 (1960), 163–88.

Church, Roy and E. M. Tansey, *Burroughs Wellcome & Co: Knowledge, trust, profit and the transformation of the British pharmaceutical industry, 1880–1940* (Lancaster, Crucible Books, 2007).

Colgrove, James, *State of immunity: The politics of vaccination in twentieth-century America* (Oakland, University of California Press, 2006).

Conrad, Peter and Kristin K. Barker, 'The social construction of illness: Key insights and policy implications', *Journal of Health and Social Behaviour*, Vol. 51, No. 1 (November 2010), S67–69.

Conrad, Peter and Joseph W. Schneider, *Deviance and medicalization: From badness to sickness* (Philadelphia, 1992).

Corcoran, Donal P., *Freedom to achieve freedom: The Irish Free State 1922–32* (Dublin, Gill & MacMillan, 2013).

Cox, Catherine and Maria Luddy (eds), *Cultures of care in Irish medical history, 1750–1970* (Basingstoke, Palgrave Macmillan, 2010).

Crawford, Margaret E., 'Typhus in nineteenth-century Ireland', in Greta Jones and Elizabeth Malcolm (eds) *Medicine, disease and the state in Ireland, 1650–1940* (Cork, Cork University Press, 1999).

Daly, Mary E., 'Death and disease in independent Ireland, c.1920–1970: A research agenda', in Catherine Cox and Maria Luddy (eds), *Cultures of care in Irish medical history, 1750–1970* (Basingstoke, Palgrave Macmillan, 2010).

Daly, Mary E., *The buffer state: The historical roots of the Department of the Environment* (Dublin, Institute of Public Administration, 1997).

Daly, Mary, 'Local appointments', in Mary E. Daly, *County & Town: One hundred years of local government in Ireland* (Dublin, Institute of Public Administration, 2001).

Deeny, James, *To cure and to care: Memoirs of a chief medical officer* (Dublin, Glendale Press, 1989).

Depypere, M., et al, 'A forgotten disease in a returning traveler from Thailand', *Acta Clinica Belgica*, Vol. 68, No. 5 (Sept–Oct 2013), 382–83.

Devereux, Eoin, 'Saving rural Ireland: Muintir na Tire and its anti-urbanism, 1931–1958', *The Canadian Journal of Irish Studies*, Vol. 17, No. 2 (December 1991), 23–30.

Diack, Leslie and David Smith, 'Professional strategies of medical officers of health in the post-war period-1: "Innovative traditionalism": the case of Dr Ian MacQueen, MOH for Aberdeen, 1952–1974, a "bull-dog" with the hide of a "rhinoceros"', *Journal of Public Health*, Vol. 24, No. 2 (2002), 123–29.

Domenech, Rosa, M. and Claudia Castaneda, 'Redefining cancer during the interwar period: British medical officers of health, state policy, managerialism, and public health', *American Journal of Public Health*, Vol. 97, No. 9 (September 2007), 1563–71.

Dwyer, Michael, 'Abandoned by God and the Corporation: housing and the health of the working class in Cork City, 1912–1924', *Saothar 38, Journal of the Irish Labour History Society* (2013), 105–18.

Dwyer, Michael, 'Cumann na nGaedheal and the reform of public health administration in the Irish Free State', *Australasian Journal of Irish Studies*, Vol. 13 (2013), 149–63.

Dwyer, Michael, 'Vaccine Trials: Dark chapter that needs answers', *Irish Examiner*, 1 December 2014.

Earner-Byrne, Lindsey, *Mother and child: Maternity and child welfare in Dublin, 1922–60* (Manchester, Manchester University Press, 2007).

Ellis, H., 'Edwin Klebs: discoverer of the bacillus of diphtheria', *British Journal of Hospital Medicine*, Vol. 74, No. 11 (Nov. 2013), 641.

Evans, Alfred S. and Philip S. Brachman (eds), *Bacterial infections of Humans: Epidemiology and control* (New York, Plenum Medical Book Co, 1998).

Farmar, Tony, *Patients, potions and physicians: A social history of medicine in Ireland* (Dublin, A & A Farmar, 2004).

Fenning, Hugh, 'The cholera epidemic in Ireland 1832–33: Priests, ministers, doctors', *Archivium Hibernicum*, Vol. 57 (2003), 77–125.

Ferriter, Diarmuid 'Local government, public health and welfare in twentieth-century Ireland', in Mary E. Daly (ed.), *County & town: One hundred years of local government in Ireland* (Dublin, Institute of Public Administration, 2001).

Foley, Caitriona, '"This revived old plague": Coping with flu', in Catherine Cox and Maria Luddy (eds) *Cultures of care in Irish medical history, 1950–1970* (Basingstoke, Palgrave Macmillan, 2010).

Foucault, Michel, (Translated by A. M. Sheridan), *The birth of the clinic: An archaeology of medical perception* (London, 2009).

Gaffney, Patrick, 'Book review of Kiely's, Text-book of Surgery', in *Medical Alumni Newsletter*, University College Cork, No. 8 (May 2010), 19.

Garcia, Vincent, 'Therapeutic accidents and new health practices. Colombian medicine in the face of the anti-diphtheria vaccination catastrophe of Medellin, 1930', *Historica Crítica*, No. 46 (January/April 2012), 110–31.

Garvin, Tom, *Preventing the future: Why was Ireland so poor for so long?* (Dublin, Gill & Macmillan, 2004).

Geary, Laurence M., '"Report upon the recent epidemic fever in Ireland": the evidence from Cork' in John Crowley, et al (eds) *Atlas of the Great Irish Famine, 1845–52* (Cork, Cork University Press, 2012).

Geary, Laurence, M., 'The 1956 polio epidemic in Cork', *History Ireland*, Vol. 14, No. 3 (2006), 34–37.

Gill, D., 'Vaccination, not vacillation', *Irish Medical Journal*, Vol. 104, No. 10 (Nov–Dec 2011), 294.

Gorsky, Martin, 'Local government health services in interwar England: Problems of quantification and interpretation', *Bulletin of the History of Medicine*, Vol. 85 (2011), 384–412.

Gorsky, Martin, 'Local leadership in public health: the role of the medical officer of health in Britain, 1872-1974', *Journal of Epidemiology and Community Health*, Vol. 61 (2007), 468–72.

Gorsky, Martin, 'Public health in inter-war Britain: Did it fail?' *Dynamis*, Vol. 28 (2008), 175–98.

Grodin and Glantz (eds), *Children as research subjects; science, ethics & law* (Oxford, Oxford University Press, 1994).

Guilfoile, Patrick, *Deadly diseases and epidemics: Diphtheria* (New York, Chelsea House, 2009).

Halliday, Stephen, 'Death and miasma in Victorian London: an obstinate belief', *British Medical Journal*, Vol. 323 (22 December 2001), 1467–71.

Hammonds, Evelynn Maxine, *Childhood's deadliest scourge: The campaign to control diphtheria in New York City, 1880–1930* (Baltimore, Johns Hopkins University Press, 1999).

Hardy, Anne, 'Review: Evelynn Maxine Hammonds, *Childhood's deadliest scourge: The campaign to control diphtheria in New York City, 1880–1930* (Baltimore, 1999)', *Medical History*, Vol. 45, No. 2 (March 2001), 297–99.

Hardy, Anne, 'Tracheotomy versus intubation: Surgical intervention in diphtheria in Europe and the United States, 1825–1930', *Bulletin of the History of Medicine* (1992), 536–59.

Hardy, Anne, *The epidemic streets: Infectious disease and the rise of preventive medicine, 1856–1900* (Oxford, Oxford University Press, 1993).

Hensey, Brendan, *The health services of Ireland* (Dublin, Institute of Public Administration, 1959).

Hobbins, Peter, '"Immunization is as popular as a death adder": The Bundaberg tragedy and the politics of medical science in interwar Australia', *Social History of Medicine*, Vol. 24, No. 2 (2011), 426–44.

Hooker, Clare and Alison Bashford, 'Diphtheria and Australian public health: Bacteriology and its complex applications, c. 1890–1930', *Medical History*, No. 46 (2002), 41–64.

Hooker, Clare, 'Diphtheria, immunization and the Bundaberg tragedy: A study of public health in Australia', *Health and History*, Vol. 2, No. 1 (July 2000), 52–57.

Horgan, John, *Noel Browne: Passionate outsider* (Dublin, Gill & Macmillan, 2000).

Horton, Richard, 'The moribund body of medical history', *The Lancet*, Vol. 384, No. 9940 (26 July 2014), 292.

Huisman, Frank and John Harley Warner (eds), *Locating medical history: The stories and their meanings* (Baltimore, Johns Hopkins University Press, 2004).

Hume, Edgar, 'Francis Home M. D. (1919–1813), The Scottish military surgeon who first described diphtheria as a clinical entity', *Bulletin of the History of Medicine* (1 Jan. 1942), 48.

Jones, Greta, 'The campaign against tuberculosis in Ireland, 1899–1914', Jones, Greta and Elizabeth Malcolm (eds), *Medicine, disease and the state in Ireland, 1650–1940* (Cork, Cork University Press, 1999).

Jones, Greta, 'The Rockefeller Foundation and medical education in Ireland in the 1920s', *Irish Historical Studies*, Vol. 30, No. 120 (Nov. 1997), 564–80.

Jones, Greta, and Elizabeth Malcolm (eds) *Medicine, disease and the state in Ireland, 1650–1940* (Cork, Cork University Press, 1999).

Jones, Greta, *Captain of all these men of death: The history of Tuberculosis in nineteenth and twentieth-century Ireland* (New York, Rodopi, 2001).

Jordan, Donald, *Land and popular politics in Ireland: County Mayo from the plantation to the land war* (Cambridge, Cambridge University Press, 1994).

Kelly, James, '"Bleeding, vomiting and purging": The medical response to ill health in eighteenth-century Ireland' in Catherine Cox and Maria Luddy, *Cultures of care in Irish medical history, 1750–1950* (Basingstoke, Palgrave Macmillan, 2010).

Kelly, Laura, 'Rickets and Irish children: Dr Ella Webb and the early work of the Children's Sunshine Home, 1925-1946', in Anne MacLellan and Alice Maugher (eds), *Growing Pains: Childhood illness in Ireland, 1750–1950* (Kildare, Irish Academic Press, 2013).

Kelly, Susan, '"And so to bed": Bone and joint tuberculosis in children in Ireland, 1920–1950', in Anne MacLellan and Alice Maugher (eds), *Growing pains: Childhood illness in Ireland*, 1750–1950 (Kildare, Irish Academic Press, 2013).

Kinealy, Christine, *A death-dealing famine: The great hunger in Ireland* (London, Pluto Press, 1997).

Knirck, Jason, *Afterimage of the revolution: Cumann na nGaedheal and Irish politics, 1922–1932* (Wisconsin, University of Wisconsin Press, 2014).

Kohn, George, *Encyclopaedia of plague and pestilence: From ancient times to the present* (New York, Infobase Publishing, 2008).

Kruse, Jutta, 'Saving Irish national infants or protecting the infant nation? Irish anti-vaccination discourse, 1900–1930', *History Studies*, Vol. 13 (2012), 91–113.

Larson, Heidi, et al, 'Addressing the vaccine confidence gap', *The Lancet*, Vol. 378, No. 9790 (6 August 2011), 526–35.

Leavitt, Judith Walzer 'Writing public health history: The need for a social scaffolding', *Reviews in American History*, Vol. 4, No. 2 (June 1976), 150–57.

Leavitt, Judith Walzer, 'Medicine in context', *American Historical Review*, Vol. 95 (December 1990), 1471–72.

Lederer, Susan, 'Children as guinea pigs: Historical perspectives', *Accountability in Research*, Vol. 10, No. 1 (2003), 1–16.

Lederer, Susan, 'Experimentation on human beings', *Organisation of American Historians Magazine of History*, Vol. 19 (2005), 20–22.

Lederer, Susan, *Subjected to science: Human experimentation in America before the Second World War* (Baltimore, Johns Hopkins University Press, 1995).

Lee, J. J., *Ireland 1912–1985: Politics and society* (Cambridge, Cambridge University Press, 1989).

Lewis, Jane, 'The prevention of diphtheria in Canada and Britain, 1914–1945', *Journal of Social History*, Vol. 20, No. 1 (Autumn 1986), 163–76.

Linton, Derek S., *Emil von Behring: Infectious disease, immunology, serum therapy* (Philadelphia, American Philosophical Society, 2005).

Lyons, J. B., 'Irish medicine's appeal to Rockefeller, 1920s', *Irish Journal of Medical Science* (January, February, March 1997), 50–56.

McCarthy, Andrew, 'Aspects of local health in Ireland in the 1950s', in Dermot Keogh et al (ed.), *The lost decade: Ireland in the 1950s* (Cork, Mercier Press, 2004).

McFarlane, Sir Frank Burnet and David O. White, *Natural history of infectious disease* (Cambridge, Cambridge University Press, 1972).

McKeown, Thomas, *The modern rise of populations* (London, Edward Arnold, 1976).

McLaurin, Susan and David Smith, 'Professional strategies of medical officers of health in the post-war period-2: "Progressive realism": the case of Dr R. J. Donaldson, MOH for Teesside, 1968-1974', *Journal of Public Health* Vol. 24, No. 2 (2002), 130–35.

MacLellan, Anne and Alice Maugher (eds), *Growing pains: Childhood illness in Ireland, 1750–1950* (Kildare, Irish Academic Press, 2013).

MacLellan, Anne, 'The Penny Test: Tuberculin testing and paediatric practice in Ireland, 1900–1960', in MacLellan, Anne, and Alice Mauger (eds), *Growing pains: Childhood illness in Ireland, 1750-1950* (Kildare, Irish Academic Press, 2013).

Marguiles, Philip, *Diphtheria* (New York, Rosen Publishing, 2005).

Meehan, Ciara, *The Cosgrave party: A history of Cumann na nGaedheal* (Dublin, Royal Irish Academy, 2010).

Menut, Phillippe, 'The Lübeck catastrophe and its consequences for anti-tuberculosis BCG vaccination', *Singular selves: Historical issues and contemporary debates in immunology.* (Paris, Elsevier, 2001).

Mitchell, Allan, 'An inexact science: the statistics of tuberculosis in late nineteenth-century France', *Social History of Medicine*, Vol. 3, No. 3 (1990), 387–403.

Mortimer, P. P., 'The diphtheria vaccine debacle of 1940 that ushered in comprehensive childhood immunization in the United Kingdom', *Epidemiology and Infection*, Vol. 139 (2001), 487–93.

Nyhan, Miriam, *Are you still below? The Ford Marina Plant, Cork, 1917–1984* (Cork, Collins Press, 2007).

Ó hÓgartaigh, Margaret, 'Dr Dorothy Price and the elimination of childhood tuberculosis', in Joost Augusteijn (ed.), *Ireland in the 1930s. New perspectives* (Dublin, Four Courts Press, 1999).

O'Brien, Joseph V., *Dear, dirty Dublin: A city in distress, 1899–1916* (Oakland, University of California Press, 1982).

O'Doherty, Mary, 'Irish medical historiography' *Irish Journal of Medical Science*, Vol. 170, No. 4 (2001), 256–60.

O'Grada, Cormac, *A rocky road: The Irish economy since the 1920s* (Manchester, Manchester University Press, 1997).

O'Halpin, Eunan, 'Politics and the State, 1922–32', in J. R. Hill (ed.), *A new history of Ireland: VII: Ireland, 1921–84* (Oxford, Oxford University Press, 2010).

Pappworth, M. H., *Human guinea pigs: Experimentation on man* (Boston, Beacon Press, 1967).

Parish, H. J., *A history of immunization* (London, E & S Livingstone, 1965).

Parish, H. J., *Victory with vaccines: The story of immunization* (London, E & S Livingstone, 1968).

Patterson, James T., 'How do we write the history of disease', *Health and History*, Vol. 1, No. 1 (1998), 5–29.

Plotkin, Stanley, A., *Mass vaccination: Global aspects-progress and obstacles* (New York, Springer, 2006).

Plotkin, Stanley, W. Orenstein and P. Offit, *Vaccines* (Elsevier, 2008).

Porter, Dorothy and Roy Porter 'The politics of prevention: Anti-vaccinationism and public health in nineteenth century England', *Medical History*, Vol. 32, No. 3 (July 1998), 231–52.

Porter, Dorothy, *Health, civilization and the state: A history of public health from ancient to modern times* (London, Routledge, 1999).

Porter, Roy, *The Cambridge illustrated history of medicine* (Cambridge, Cambridge University Press, 1996).

Porter, Roy, *The greatest benefit to mankind: a medical history of humanity from antiquity to the present* (London, Harper Collins, 1997).

Purdue, Olwen, 'The Irish Poor Law in a north Antrim town, 1861–1921', *Irish Historical Studies*, Vol. XXXVII, No. 148 (November 2011), 567–83.

Regan, John M., *Countering the revolutionaries: An examination of the Cumann na nGaedheal party 1922–25* (Belfast, Queens University of Belfast, 1994).

Robins, Joseph, *The miasma: Epidemic and panic in nineteenth-century Ireland* (Dublin, Institute of Public Administration, 1995).
Roelcke, Volker and Giovanni Maio (eds), *Twentieth century ethics of human subjects research: Historical perspectives on values, practices, and regulations* (München, Franz Steiner Verlag, 2004).
Rosen, George, *A history of public health* (Baltimore, Johns Hopkins University Press, 2003).
Rosenberg, Charles E. and Rosemary Stevens (ed.) *History and health policy in the United States: Putting the past back in* (New Jersey, Rutgers University Press, 2006).
Rosenberg, Charles E., *Explaining epidemics and other studies in the history of medicine* (Cambridge, Cambridge University Press, 1992).
Rosenberg, Charles E., *The cholera years: The United States in 1832, 1849 and 1866* (Chicago, University of Chicago Press, 1962).
Rothman, Davis, 'Ethics and human experimentation', *New England Medical Journal*, Vol. 317, No. 19 (1987), 1195–99.
Rothstein, William G., *Public health and the risk factor: A history of an uneven medical revolution* (New York, University of Rochester Press, 2003).
Sigerist, Henry, 'The history of medicine and the history of disease', *Bulletin of the Institute of the History of Medicine*, Vol. 4 (1936), 1–13.
Welshman, John, 'The Medical Officer of Health in England and Wales, 1900–1974: watchdog or lapdog?' *Journal of Public Health Medicine*, Vol. 19, No. 4 (1997), 443–50.
Welshman, John, *Municipal medicine: Public health in twentieth-century Britain* (Oxford, Peter Lang, 2000).
Whitfield, A. G. W., 'The kiss of death', *Annals of the Royal College of Surgeons of England*, Vol. 61, No. 5 (September 1979), 390–92.

Electronic Resources

Central Statistics Office, *Annual reports on marriages, births, and deaths in Ireland 1864–1964*, http://www.cso.ie/en/releasesandpublications/birthsdeathsandmarriages/archive/annualreportsonmarriagesbirthsanddeathsinirelandfrom1864to2000/.
Control of Clinical Trials Act, 1987. http://www.irishstatutebook.ie/1987/en/act/pub/0028/index.html.
Control of Clinical Trials and Drugs Act, 1990. http://www.irishstatutebook.ie/1990/en/act/pub/0017/.
Dáil Éireann, *Select committee on the health services* (1962). http://www.lenus.ie/hse/bitstream/10147/238558/1/SelectCommitteOnTheHealthServices.pdf.
DCYA http://www.dcya.gov.ie/documents/Mother_and_Baby_Homes/20150109Draft OrderCommofInvestigation.pdf.
Department of Children and Youth Affairs, Commission of Investigation (Mother and Baby Homes and certain related matters) Order 2015, Section I, (V): 9 January 2015.
European Centre for Disease 'A historical perspective', *Prevention and Control, Scientific panel on childhood immunization schedule: Diphtheria-tetanus-pertussis (DTP) vaccination*. http://www.ecdc.europa.eu/en/publications/Publications/0911_GUI_Scientific_Panel_on_Childhood_Immunization_DTP.pdf.

Health Service Executive (HSE), 'Immunization uptake report for Ireland', *Health Protection Surveillance Centre*, Q4 2015. http://www.hpsc.ie/A-Z/VaccinePreventable/ Vaccination/ImmunizationUptakeStatistics/Immunizationuptakestatisticsat12and 24monthsofage/QuarterlyReports/2013/File,14514,en.pdf.

Health Service Executive (HSE), 'Protect, Prevent, Immunise' (Last updated 13 November 2013). http://www.immunization.ie/en/ChildhoodImmunization/Primary ImmunizationSchedule/.

Health Service Executive (HSE), http://www.hpsc.ie/A-Z/VaccinePreventable/ Diphtheria/Factsheets/DiphtheriaFrequentlyAskedQuestions/.

Health Service Executive (HSE). http://www.immunization.ie/en/EXTRADOWN LOADS/Text_15414_en.html.

Houses of the Oireachtas, Dáil Debates. http://debates.oireachtas.ie/dail/.

Irish Council for Bioethics, 'Operational procedures for research ethics committees' http://www.dohc.ie/working_groups/Current/nacb/Operational_Procedures.pdf? direct=1.

Lyons, Declan, 'Medicine in Limerick in the 20th Century' (2008). http://www.3bv. org/wp-content/themes/3bv/downloads/MEDICINE-IN-LIMERICK.pdf.

Nyhan, Brendan, et al, 'Effective messages in vaccine promotion: A randomised trial', *Paediatrics*, 3 March, 2014. http://pediatrics.aappublications.org/content/ early/2014/02/25/peds.2013-2365.

Royal College of Physicians, 'National BCG Committee'. http://rcpilibrary.blogspot. ie/2010/08/national-bcg-committee-ireland.html.

UNICEF, World Health Organization, The World Bank, *State of the world's vaccines and immunization*, 3rd ed. (Geneva, 2009). http://www.unicef.org/media/files/ SOWVI_full_report_english_LR1.pdf.

World Health Organization, 'Diptheria reported cases' (updated 6 September 2017). http://apps.who.int/immunization_monitoring/globalsummary/timeseries/tsinci- dencediphtheria.html.

World Health Organization, 'Immunization, vaccines and biologicals' (updated 17 July 2014). http://www.who.int/immunization/en/.

World Health Organization, Draft Twelfth WHO General Programme of Work: Draft for discussion by the Executive Board in January 2013, http://apps.who.int/gb/ ebwha/pdf_files/EB132/B132_26-en.pdf?ua=1.

Unpublished Theses

Breslin, Suzanne, 'The quiet exception to every rule': The motivations and tensions behind the diphtheria immunization scheme in Dublin, 1929–1948. Unpublished MA thesis, School of History and Archives, University College Dublin, August 2012.

Grimes, Thomas, 'Starting Ireland on the road to industry: Henry Ford in Cork', Unpublished PhD thesis, National University of Ireland, Galway, 2008.

MacLellan, Anne, *That 'preventable and curable disease': Dr Dorothy Price and the eradication of tuberculosis in Ireland, 1930–1960*. Unpublished PhD thesis, School of History and Archives, University College Dublin, August 2011.

Index

Printed and bound by CPI Group (UK) Ltd, Croydon, CR0 4YY

27/10/2024

14580407-0004